MW00825371

Renal Diet Cookbook for Caregivers

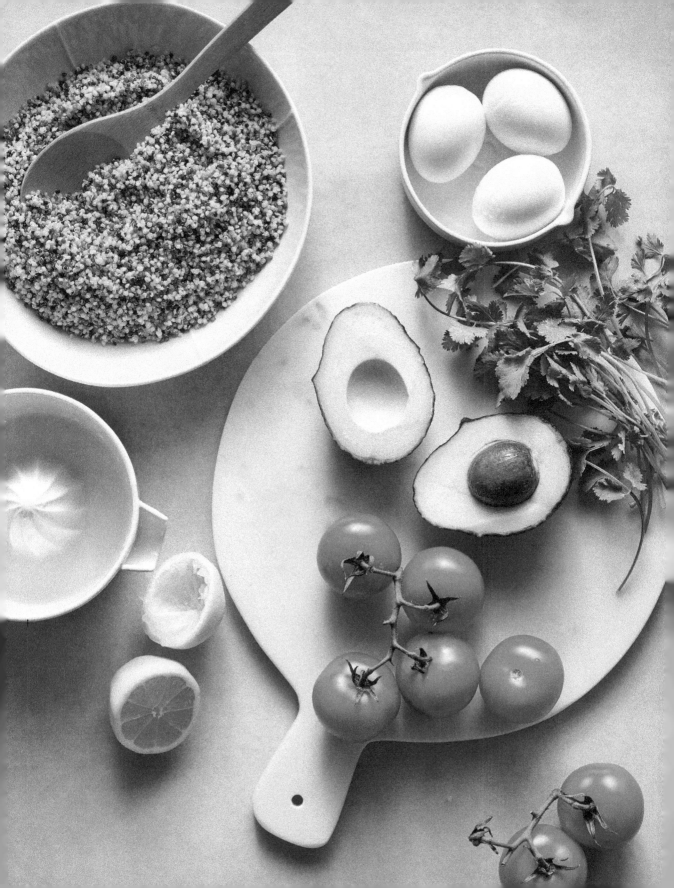

Renal Diet
Cookbook for
Caregivers

Recipes, Tips, and Meal Plans to Manage
Kidney Disease Together

Emily Campbell, RD, CDE, MScFN

ROCKRIDGE
PRESS

Copyright © 2022 by Rockridge Press, Oakland, California

No part of this publication may be reproduced, stored in a retrieval system, or transmitted in any form or by any means, electronic, mechanical, photocopying, recording, scanning, or otherwise, except as permitted under Sections 107 or 108 of the 1976 United States Copyright Act, without the prior written permission of the Publisher. Requests to the Publisher for permission should be addressed to the Permissions Department, Rockridge Press, 1955 Broadway, Suite 400, Oakland, CA 94612.

Limit of Liability/Disclaimer of Warranty: The Publisher and the author make no representations or warranties with respect to the accuracy or completeness of the contents of this work and specifically disclaim all warranties, including without limitation warranties of fitness for a particular purpose. No warranty may be created or extended by sales or promotional materials. The advice and strategies contained herein may not be suitable for every situation. This work is sold with the understanding that the Publisher is not engaged in rendering medical, legal, or other professional advice or services. If professional assistance is required, the services of a competent professional person should be sought. Neither the Publisher nor the author shall be liable for damages arising herefrom. The fact that an individual, organization, or website is referred to in this work as a citation and/or potential source of further information does not mean that the author or the Publisher endorses the information the individual, organization, or website may provide or recommendations they/it may make. Further, readers should be aware that websites listed in this work may have changed or disappeared between when this work was written and when it is read.

For general information on our other products and services or to obtain technical support, please contact our Customer Care Department within the United States at (866) 744-2665, or outside the United States at (510) 253-0500.

Rockridge Press publishes its books in a variety of electronic and print formats. Some content that appears in print may not be available in electronic books, and vice versa.

TRADEMARKS: Rockridge Press and the Rockridge Press logo are trademarks or registered trademarks of Callisto Media Inc. and/or its affiliates, in the United States and other countries, and may not be used without written permission. All other trademarks are the property of their respective owners. Rockridge Press is not associated with any product or vendor mentioned in this book.

Interior and Cover Designer: Scott Petrower
Art Producer: Samantha Ulban
Editor: Rebecca Markley
Production Manager: Riley Hoffman
Production Editor: Melissa Edeburn

Photography © 2021 Marija Vidal, cover and 82; © Antonis Achilleos, pp. ii, x; StockFood / Bauer Syndication; pp. vi, 50; © Elysa Weitala, p. viii; © Nadine Greeff, pp. 19, 140; Martí Sans/ Stocksy, p. 20; © Darren Muir, pp. 34, 139; StockFood / The Picture Pantry, pp. 40, 98; StockFood / Zouev, Tanya, p. 110. Food Styling by Victoria Woollard, cover.

Author photo courtesy of Amanda Lee – SimpleeCreatives.

Paperback ISBN: 978-1-64876-548-3 | eBook ISBN: 978-1-64876-549-0
R0

This book is meant to inspire anyone
who has ever thought a renal diet
meant avoiding your favorite foods.

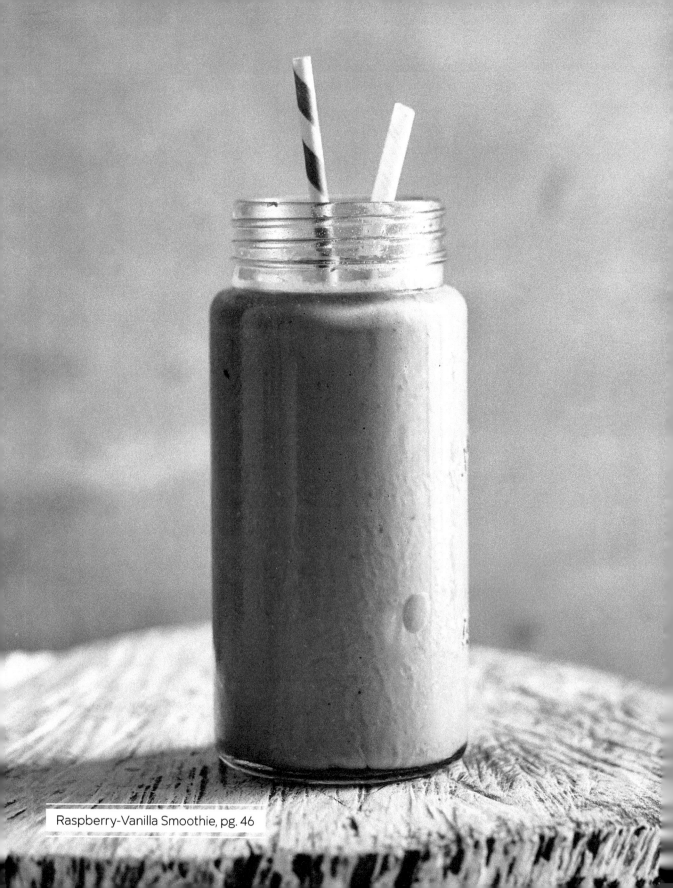

Raspberry-Vanilla Smoothie, pg. 46

Contents

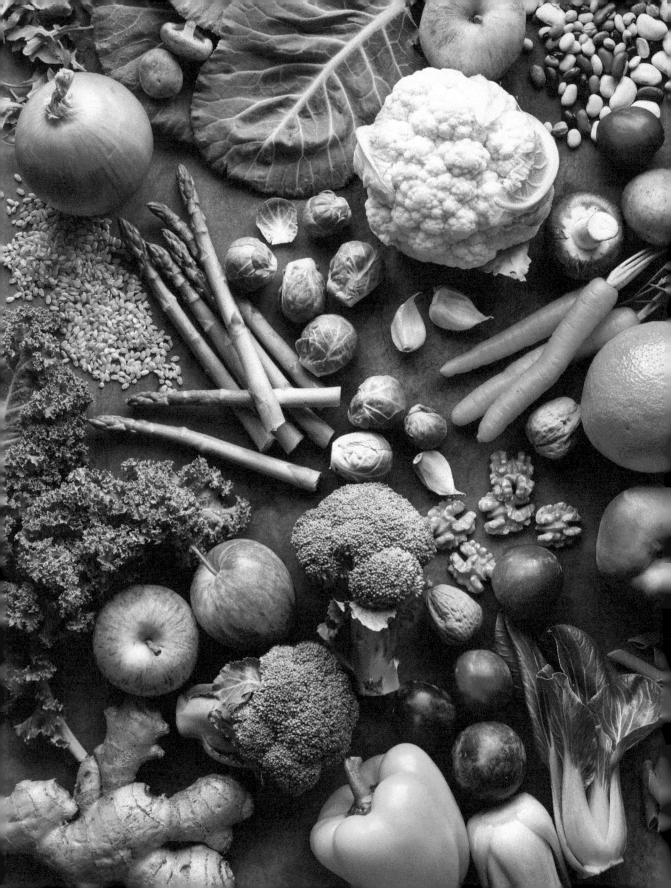

Introduction

According to the National Kidney Foundation, chronic kidney disease (CKD) affects one in seven in the United States, or some 30 million people, most of whom are unaware that they are living with the disease. You and your loved one are not alone on the CKD journey.

Your loved one may have been given the recommendation to follow a kidney-friendly diet, and as a caregiver, you may feel confused by or frustrated with all the nutrient and nutrition requirements. My hope is that after reading this book, you will feel more confident and inspired to prepare delicious and nutritious meals for your loved one and yourself. As a registered dietitian and certified diabetes educator, I have seen the impact nutrition can have on improving quality of life. This book can support you as a caregiver with evidence-based nutrition recommendations and recipes that will take the stress of providing good nutrition off your plate and give you peace of mind that the meals you are preparing can help delay the progression of CKD.

This book was designed to help you and your loved one understand how to plan balanced meals that are kidney-friendly for every stage of CKD. It includes 75 recipes that are labeled for each stage of CKD, along with nutritional information focused on CKD-relevant nutrients: sodium, protein, potassium, and phosphorus. I hope these recipes inspire you to try new foods that are not just nutritious, but also enjoyable to eat.

Please note that the contents of this book should not be taken as medical advice and are not meant to be a substitute for the medical advice provided to you or your loved one by a doctor or dietitian. Before embarking on any new eating plan, it's best to consult with your loved one's healthcare provider.

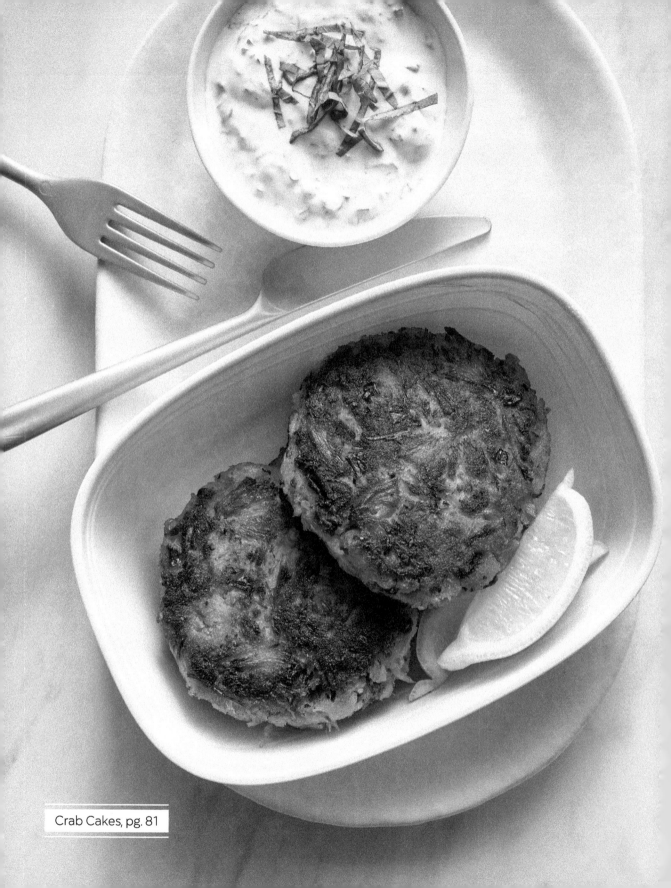

Crab Cakes, pg. 81

CHAPTER ONE

A Caregiver's Guide to the Renal Diet

One of the best ways you can support your loved one is to learn and be informed about CKD. This chapter covers the basics of chronic kidney disease. You will learn what to expect at each stage of the disease and discover strategies for preparing meals. The renal diet is often viewed as difficult to follow because of its emphasis on many important nutrients; however, supporting your loved one's nutrition does not need to be complicated anymore.

Chronic Kidney Disease and Your Loved One

Your loved one is not alone on their CKD journey: The National Institute of Diabetes and Digestive and Kidney Diseases estimates that more than 30 million Americans have CKD. To help support your loved one, you need to understand the role of the kidneys.

The kidneys are two bean-shaped organs located on the back of the body, underneath the rib cage on both sides. They are important for filtering waste and removing excess fluid from the body. The kidneys also play an important role in regulating blood pressure, keeping bones healthy, and assisting with red blood cell production; as a result, your loved one may develop other health conditions, such as anemia or weakened bones, because of their kidney disease. Individuals with CKD have decreased kidney function, so waste products (such as urea, uric acid, and creatinine, among others) as well as some electrolytes (potassium or phosphorus, for example) begin to build up in the blood according to the US Centers for Disease Control and Prevention (CDC).

There are five stages of CKD, which are measured by the Estimated Glomerular Filtration Rate (eGFR), a percentage value that indicates the level of kidney function. The lower the eGFR, the lower the kidney function. As kidney function declines, waste products begin to accumulate in the blood, and other symptoms, such as loss of appetite, fatigue, swelling in hands or feet, urinating less frequently, and itching, may appear as a result.

The risk of developing CKD increases as we age, especially after age 60. CKD is a progressive disease, which means that kidney function declines over time. CKD is commonly associated with other conditions such as diabetes, high blood pressure, and heart disease. Although CKD is not completely reversible, the progression of the disease or further kidney damage can be delayed, and nutrition plays an important role in this. By taking steps such as limiting sodium and protein, meeting potassium and phosphorus requirements, and managing other conditions associated with CKD, such as diabetes or high blood pressure, your loved one can exert control over how hard their kidneys are working and help preserve the function of these vital organs.

As always, make sure to work in conjunction with your loved one's healthcare team before embarking on a new way of eating.

WHERE TO START?

Getting started with caring for your loved one with CKD can be overwhelming—there's a lot to learn and to prepare. This book aims to simplify the process and support you and your loved one on their health journey. Here are some tips on where to start as a caregiver:

Learn as much as you can about the condition. Knowledge is power—start by learning about CKD through the National Kidney Foundation (kidney.org) or the Kidney Foundation of Canada (kidney.ca). These organizations provide credible information about CKD, from the basics of CKD to living with CKD and beyond, as well as offer free webinars and resources to support you and your loved one.

Seek financial assistance if you need it. If your loved one can't afford healthcare expenses associated with CKD, speak with the social worker on their healthcare team or seek out financial assistance programs through organizations such as the American Kidney Fund or the Kidney Foundation of Canada.

Be both positive—and realistic. With a new diagnosis, adjusting to a new lifestyle or supporting a loved one with CKD may feel overwhelming. Build a foundation for a positive attitude: take it one day at a time and do small things, like saying thank you and remaining grateful for what you do have. You may even want to keep a gratitude journal to take pleasure in good experiences. This has been shown to increase positivity. Keep an open mind and learn as much as you can about CKD to help you stay realistic.

Find support. Join a support group through the National Kidney Foundation or the Kidney Foundation of Canada to meet other caregivers. Having a larger support system can help you and your loved one adjust to new routines, continue to learn, and feel less alone in the process.

Keep a journal of notes and questions. While you are learning, take notes and write down questions to ask your loved one's healthcare team at your next meeting. Learn how to advocate for your loved one in the next section (page 21).

What to Expect Stage by Stage

There are many causes of CKD, such as diabetes, high blood pressure, and genetic or autoimmune disorders. CKD is a progressive disease, meaning the loss of function is slow and gradual and takes place over the course of months or years. The five stages of CKD are measured by the eGFR, a percentage that tells your loved one (and their healthcare team) how well their kidneys are working. In the early stages of CKD, there may be no symptoms of kidney damage or loss of function; as the disease advances, your loved one may experience symptoms. Nutrition plays an important role in managing kidney disease, because with the right nutrition changes and diet choices for each stage, the kidneys have less waste to filter and their function can be preserved. Nutrition also helps manage lab values for electrolytes at later stages. Understanding your loved one's stage of kidney disease helps empower you to ask their kidney team questions and make appropriate nutrition changes.

Stage 1

Slight kidney damage with normal or increased filtration (eGFR > 90 mL/min/1.73m^2)

Stage 1 CKD is considered mild kidney damage, with the eGFR at 90 or greater. Although the kidneys appear to be functioning normally, the kidney team will see changes in the blood or urine. Most people have not been diagnosed at this stage because they are asymptomatic, meaning they are peeing normally, have no waste products accumulating in the body, and exhibit no symptoms like shortness of breath or swelling in the legs or feet.

Stage 2

Mild decrease in kidney function (eGFR = 60–89 mL/min/1.73m^2)

In stage 2 CKD, the eGFR will decrease to between 60 and 89 as your loved one's kidney function declines. This stage is often referred to as mildly decreased function, because individuals may continue to be asymptomatic. The typical functions of the kidneys are maintained, and electrolytes, such as potassium and phosphorus, remain normal.

Stage 3

Moderate decrease in kidney function (eGFR = 30–59 mL/min/1.73m^2)

Stage 3 CKD is moderate kidney damage. As kidney function declines, waste products build up because the kidneys are unable to eliminate them. This is called *uremia*. Symptoms of uremia are nausea, vomiting, decreased appetite, and confusion. Other common symptoms in stage 3 include fatigue; swelling in the hands or feet due to fluid retention; shortness of breath; peeing less frequently; changes in urine color (may be foamy, dark orange, brown or tea color, and concentrated); back pain where the kidneys are located; sleep problems; and muscle cramps or restless legs. Typically, at this stage, your loved one will be referred to a nephrologist (a doctor who specializes in treating kidney disease) as well as a dietitian. If your loved one's doctor has not referred them to a nephrology team, ask for a referral.

Stage 4

Severe decrease in kidney function (eGFR = 15–29 mL/min/1.73m^2)

With stage 4 CKD, the eGFR is between 15 and 29, which means the kidneys are moderately or severely damaged. At this stage, your loved one may have symptoms such as swelling in their extremities, back pain, or peeing more or less than normal, and is more likely to develop complications from CKD, such as high blood pressure, anemia, a buildup of electrolytes in the blood, and bone disease. Medication changes for diabetes and high blood pressure may be stopped or started to help preserve kidney function. At this stage, it is important to speak with your loved one's healthcare team about how to prepare for kidney failure. When the kidneys have failed, renal replacement therapy (such as dialysis or a kidney transplant) will be necessary.

Stage 5

Kidney failure/end-stage CKD (eGFR < 15 mL/min/1.73m^2)

Stage 5 CKD means the eGFR is less than 15 and the kidneys are getting very close to failing—or have failed. When the kidneys fail, waste products build up in the blood, which can make your loved one sick. Some common symptoms of kidney failure include itching, muscle cramps, nausea or vomiting, lack of appetite, swelling, and difficulty breathing. These symptoms occur because of the accumulation of waste products in the body. When the kidneys have failed, dialysis or a kidney transplant is necessary to stay alive. There are two types of dialysis: hemodialysis, in which a machine called a *dialyzer* filters waste and excess fluid from the blood; and peritoneal dialysis, in which a catheter is inserted into the abdominal cavity and a dialysis solution is used to remove waste and excess fluid through filling and draining this solution in the abdominal cavity. Your loved one's healthcare team can support you in preparing for dialysis or a kidney transplant.

Renal Diet 101

In this section, you will find an overview of the nutrition guidelines for each stage of CKD. Proper nutrition can help preserve kidney function by giving the kidneys fewer waste products to filter. We'll look at the common nutrients in the CKD diet and break them down by stage to help you understand how much of certain foods your loved one should consume, and how often, depending on their stage of CKD. This book includes dietary guidelines and meal plans for individuals with CKD stages 1 to 3, stage 4, and stage 5 (dialysis). In the food lists on page 122, you will find a list of common foods and their nutritional information. Remember, though, that it is important to speak with your loved one's healthcare team to discuss their individual nutrition needs.

Key Nutrients

Monitoring key nutrients is imperative on a CKD diet, and depending on your loved one's stage of CKD, there may be specific nutrients to avoid. Here is a breakdown.

POTASSIUM

Potassium plays an important role in helping our heart beat, and too much or too little potassium can be dangerous. A low-potassium or potassium-restricted diet is only necessary if potassium lab values exceed 5.0 mmol/L in **stage 1 to 3** (or 5.5 mmol/L in **stage 5, if on dialysis),** as this may cause an irregular heartbeat. Potassium restrictions are not common in stages 1 to 3, as the kidneys are still able to filter potassium through the urine. If your loved one is instructed to follow a low-potassium plan, limit potassium to 2,000 mg or less per day by choosing low-potassium foods (foods with more than 200 mg per ½-cup serving are considered high-potassium foods). Use the food lists on page 122 as a resource for high- and low-potassium foods. Some individuals may have

SUPPORTING YOUR LOVED ONE

Being a caregiver is a challenging and rewarding role. You know your loved one best, so trust your instincts. This section will provide you with strategies and tips for supporting your loved one as a caregiver.

Advocating for Their Needs

Healthcare appointments can be overwhelming, but knowing the right questions to ask or supportive things to say can make a big difference. Here are some ways you can advocate for your loved one with their healthcare team:

Learn as much as you can. Understanding your loved one's condition and how to care for it is important. You'll feel less anxiety and be more effective as a caregiver when you're armed with information.

Take notes and track symptoms. Having a journal or notebook where you can write down medical questions or symptoms that come up between appointments is important. This will help you provide the healthcare team with more information about your loved one's condition.

Keep track of questions you want to ask. Going to appointments with questions written down can help decrease stress and allow you to participate more in the appointment. Here are some questions to ask your loved one's healthcare team:

1. What is my loved one's stage of CKD?
2. How many grams of protein are appropriate per day?
3. How many ounces of fluid are needed?
4. Does potassium need to be restricted?
5. Is a nutritional supplement or multivitamin needed?

Follow up on test results. When caregivers have copies of test results, it is easier to make sure that all doctors have the right information (especially if an emergency room or urgent care visit occurs). As a caregiver, your loved one's test results can also help you learn more about their medical condition and health trends.

continued ▶

Advocate for kidney patients. As a caregiver, your voice is powerful in supporting your loved one as well as others living with CKD. And advocating for those living with CKD is important to help improve access to resources and healthcare. Learn more about how you can help through the American Kidney Foundation's advocacy network.

Small Ways to Show Support

These tips may seem small, but their effect can be impactful over time. When offering support to your loved one, be persistent and ask specific questions.

Instead of asking how they are, ask them if they're able to eat anything. With CKD, patients may experience a reduced appetite and may not be interested in eating. Offering snacks or having prepared meals available is a great way to show support.

Encourage social interactions. Personal visits with friends can improve well-being and help your loved one cope with their illness. Your loved one may have mobility issues, which can be a large barrier in social interactions. By hosting personal visits at home, you can support your loved one mentally—and physically.

Provide distractions. Sometimes, a bit of normalcy is the best thing you can offer as a caregiver. Look for activities you and your loved one can do together, like watching TV shows, gardening, washing the dishes, or folding the laundry.

Take "the ask" off their plate. Instead of asking what they need, be proactive and take things off their to-do list, like making sure their bills are paid or arranging a ride to their next appointment.

Don't take it personally. Everyone deals with CKD differently: some people may be willing to talk about it, others may not. Try to be comfortable with silence; it may be just what your loved one needs.

low potassium, meaning their lab values are below 3.5 mmol/L, which is also dangerous for the heart. It is important to maintain a potassium lab value from 3.5 to 5.0 mmol/L to keep your heart beating regularly.

PHOSPHORUS

With CKD, phosphorus can build up in the body, causing weak bones and hardened blood vessels. There are two sources of phosphorus: natural phosphorus and phosphorus additives. Natural phosphorus comes from foods such as animal- and plant-based proteins, dairy, nuts, and chocolate; phosphorus additives are commonly found in processed foods. It is important to avoid added phosphorus regardless of the CKD stage. Reading food labels can help you identify sources of phosphorus additives by looking for chemicals that include "phos" in their names. Too much phosphorus can cause weak bones; as your kidney function changes, your blood phosphorus may rise (this is most common in **stage 4 or 5**). When lab values exceed 1.45 mmol/L, the bones can become weak and blood vessels harden. Limiting phosphorus intake to 1,000 mg per day can help control phosphorus. Avoid high-phosphorus foods, such as cola, dairy products, organ meats, processed foods, and chocolate, as well as phosphorus additives.

PROTEIN

Protein is an important macronutrient used by the body to build muscle and fight infection. But too much protein can cause waste products to build up in the blood, making it hard for the kidneys to remove the waste when filtering. Following a low-protein diet can protect the kidneys by lightening the load they need to filter. Low-protein diets (0.6 to 0.8 grams per kilogram of body weight for those in **stage 1 or 2** or individuals at any stage who also have diabetes, or 0.55 to 0.6 grams per kilogram of body weight for those who do not have diabetes in **stages 3 to 5**) should be supervised by a registered dietitian to prevent malnutrition. Choose plant-based proteins—such as tofu, legumes or beans, nuts or nut butter—as often as possible to preserve kidney function; the organs need to do less work to filter these types of proteins. For individuals on dialysis, a higher-protein diet is needed because protein is lost during treatment. Spacing protein consumption over the course of three meals throughout the day helps lessen the load on the kidneys. Aim for 1.0 to 1.2 grams per kilogram of body weight in **stage 5 on dialysis;** this helps to preserve muscle mass.

SODIUM

Too much sodium or added salt can lead to high blood pressure and swelling in the hands or feet because the kidneys are unable to get rid of the excess fluid in the body. Limiting sodium intake to 2,300 mg per day can help. Reading food labels for low-sodium products (aim for 200 mg or less per serving) and adding flavor to meals by cooking with aromatic ingredients like garlic, onion, herbs, and spices instead of adding salt can help meet this guideline.

CARBOHYDRATES

Carbohydrates provide the body with a quick energy source and fiber. Fiber is important for managing cholesterol and blood glucose levels in diabetes, as well as preventing constipation. Plan meals that include whole grains (e.g., whole grain bread, brown rice) as often as possible. Constipation is common for those with kidney disease, especially when fluid restriction is added. Including whole grains and high-fiber foods for as long as possible can help manage constipation. Aim for 20 to 30 grams of fiber a day; choose high-fiber foods, include 2 cups of vegetables (fresh, frozen, or canned, with no added salt or sugar) per meal, and serve fruit as a snack. Depending on your loved one's potassium or phosphorus restriction, their healthcare team may provide alternative recommendations.

FATS

Choose foods with unsaturated fats and omega-3 fatty acids, such as nuts (e.g., almonds or walnuts), seeds (e.g., pumpkin), olive or canola oil, or fatty fish (e.g., salmon). These foods help increase good cholesterol in the blood. Reducing cardiovascular problems such as high cholesterol, which is associated with CKD, is important and can be done through diet. Limit saturated fat from animal-based products (e.g., fatty meats or dairy) and avoid trans fats from processed foods, as these may increase cholesterol.

Fluids

Fluids include water, coffee and tea, juice, soup, ice cream, yogurt—basically, anything that becomes liquid at room temperature. Maintaining hydration is important to help preserve kidney function, so aim for 1.5 to 2 liters of fluid per day in **stages 1 to 4,** unless a doctor has recommended a different value because of a heart condition or swelling. As kidney function declines, excessive fluid intake can be dangerous, as the fluid may accumulate in the body and lead to swelling of feet or ankles and shortness of breath. For those in **stage 5** on hemodialysis, limit fluid to urine output plus 1 liter; those on peritoneal dialysis may not need to restrict fluids, as their dialysis occurs more frequently.

Vitamins and Supplements

Vitamins and supplements can help general health and are needed for overall body function. Don't hesitate to ask your loved one's healthcare team if a supplement is needed in **stages 1 to 4**. A kidney-safe multivitamin may be recommended by the healthcare team to help prevent or treat micronutrient deficiencies in **stage 5**. Some probiotic supplements have been shown to delay the progression of kidney disease. Be sure to speak with your loved one's healthcare team before introducing supplements.

Portion Control

Part of managing your loved one's nutrition includes looking at their daily intake of macronutrients (carbohydrates, proteins, and fat) and micronutrients (vitamins and minerals). This means managing their serving sizes. Enjoying a variety of kidney-friendly foods is important to help manage CKD and preserve kidney function. At meals, aim for vegetables to take up half the plate, protein to take up one-quarter, and carbohydrates to take up the remaining one-quarter. Also plan on three meals per day, spaced no more than 4 to 6 hours apart. If meals happen at longer intervals or your loved one is hungry between meals, include a snack with fruit. Focusing on a balanced plate and spacing out meals (and protein consumption) throughout the day helps lighten the protein load on the kidneys, meaning they work less, while also meeting macronutrient and micronutrient needs for the day.

Calorie Intake

Getting enough calories is important for preventing weight loss and malnutrition. Your loved one may be at risk of losing weight with CKD because of taste changes, poor appetite, poorly planned meals, or calorie and nutrient restrictions associated with a low-protein diet. Aim for 25 to 35 calories per kilogram of body weight per day to meet energy needs. If maintaining body weight becomes a challenge, work with a registered dietitian to create a personalized plan.

To calculate your loved one's daily calorie needs, multiply their weight in kilograms by 25 and 35; this gives you the range of calories they'll need to consume to meet their body's energy needs. To calculate weight in kilograms, divide their weight in pounds by 2.2. For example, an individual who weighs 150 pounds (68.2 kilograms) requires 1,705 to 2,046 calories per day (68.2 kg x 25 calories/kg = 1,705 calories; 68.2 kg x 30 calories/kg = 2,046 calories). If your loved one is losing weight, aim to include an additional 500 calories per day for weight gain.

Considering Associated Conditions

Diabetes, high blood pressure, and heart disease are commonly found in conjunction with CKD. CKD can also develop from years of uncontrolled diabetes, high blood pressure, or high cholesterol levels. If your loved one has one or several of these conditions, it is important to manage them as well to help slow the progression of their kidney disease. Research shows that following a Mediterranean, DASH (Dietary Approaches to Stop Hypertension), or plant-based diet can be helpful in managing these conditions together. Many of the recipes in this book are suitable for those with diabetes, high blood pressure, or heart disease or include tips for adjusting to accommodate these conditions.

Here are some tips for modifying recipes to accommodate these conditions.

Diabetes

◆ Limit added sugars (honey, sugar, maple syrup, agave) in recipes. Instead, sweeten with fruit purees like unsweetened applesauce or mashed banana.

◆ Choose low-glycemic-index carbohydrates with fiber, such as parboiled rice or brown rice instead of white rice, as these do not cause blood glucose levels to rise as quickly or as high.

◆ At all meals, aim to fill half the plate with vegetables, whether fresh, frozen, or canned (with no added salt).

◆ Make water the beverage of choice.

High Blood Pressure

- Read food labels for low-sodium options. Aim for 200 mg per serving for packaged foods.

- Choose no-added-salt (sometimes shortened to "NAS" or "NSA") canned products.

- Season foods with fresh or dried herbs instead of salt.

- At all meals, aim to fill half the plate with vegetables, whether fresh, frozen, or canned (with no added salt).

Heart Disease

- Cook with heart-healthy fats, such as olive or canola oil or plant-sterol-enriched margarine, instead of butter or lard.

- Incorporate plant-based proteins. Try swapping lentils for ground beef in pasta sauce or tofu for chicken in a stir-fry.

- Aim for 3 servings per week of heart-healthy fish, such as salmon or trout.

- Choose whole grain or low-glycemic-index carbohydrates.

GLYCEMIC INDEX

The glycemic index is a measure of how quickly foods cause blood glucose levels to rise. Some foods, including as white bread, white rice, potatoes, and overripe bananas, have a higher glycemic index—meaning they cause blood glucose to rise quickly or to high levels. Foods that have a low glycemic index, such as oatmeal, sourdough bread, sweet potatoes, apples, and berries, can help control blood glucose levels.

Preparing a Kidney-Friendly Kitchen

Preparing kidney-friendly meals for your loved one does not need to be complicated. Having the right equipment available can make your life easier when cooking—and you likely already have many of the items in your kitchen.

Equipment and Tools

Here you'll find the main kitchen equipment and tools you'll need to prepare the recipes in this book.

Baking pans and dishes: Used for baking or roasting foods. This book uses a baking sheet, muffin tin, 9-by-13-inch baking dish, 8- and 9-inch square baking dishes, and a 9-inch pie plate.

Knife: Having a sharp, durable knife can make all the difference when chopping and preparing foods.

Nonstick cookware: Food does not adhere to nonstick cookware, making it less likely to burn as easily, and nonstick pans are a breeze to clean afterward. Consider investing in a few different-size skillets or sauté pans and saucepans when stocking your kitchen.

Mason jars: These come in a variety of sizes and are great for storing leftovers and quick-pickling foods.

High-speed blender: This kitchen staple is great for mixing and blending foods and for making smoothies and sauces.

Food processor: Food processors are a great tool for chopping, mixing, and pureeing foods, and even for making pie dough.

Potato masher: This gadget is great for mashing, softening, and crushing foods—and not just potatoes. A masher is ideal for breaking down chickpeas and other beans, too.

Pantry Essentials

Building your pantry can help make recipe preparation easy. The following items are basic and versatile staples that are used frequently and have a long shelf life, so keeping them on hand will make cooking easier and more efficient. The recipes in this cookbook are based on 30 pantry items that you will use repeatedly as you prepare kidney-friendly meals. Don't worry about having every item on this list right away; just choose a few recipes in the book to start and build your pantry over time.

- ☐ All-purpose flour
- ☐ Baking soda
- ☐ Black beans, canned, no-added-salt
- ☐ Broth, vegetable, no-added-salt
- ☐ Chia seeds
- ☐ Chickpeas, canned, no-added-salt
- ☐ Chocolate chips, dark, mini
- ☐ Cinnamon
- ☐ Cocoa powder, unsweetened
- ☐ Cornstarch
- ☐ Cream of tartar
- ☐ Cumin
- ☐ Dill, dried
- ☐ Garlic powder
- ☐ Honey

- ☐ Oats, rolled (old-fashioned)
- ☐ Olive oil
- ☐ Onion powder
- ☐ Oregano
- ☐ Orzo
- ☐ Paprika
- ☐ Rice, parboiled
- ☐ Red pepper flakes
- ☐ Soy sauce, low-sodium
- ☐ Sugar, white
- ☐ Tahini
- ☐ Vanilla extract
- ☐ Vinegar, apple cider
- ☐ Vinegar, red wine
- ☐ Yeast, instant

WHEN YOU NEED A BREAK FROM COOKING

Sometimes you might be tired of cooking, you might not have the energy to cook, or you might be short on time. Here are some tips for serving up nutritious, kidney-friendly meals when you need a time-out from cooking.

Batch cook and freeze meals for emergencies. Prepare a large batch of full meals and refrigerate or freeze portions to serve later. Having on hand airtight containers with tight-fitting lids made from materials that freeze well makes batch cooking easy. Being organized with containers lowers stress when meal prepping and prevents big messes in the kitchen or freezer.

Ask for help from your support system. Having a support system is important. Asking for and accepting meals from your support system is not always easy, but seeking help has been linked to better health outcomes. Being specific about the support you need may make it easier to ask for help and rally the troops when you are in need.

Check out healthy meal-delivery services. Meal-delivery services can be a convenient way of getting balanced meals that are ready to cook. Before ordering, review the menu online or in person, and look for low-sodium options or ask the company if they have any kidney-friendly options. Some companies cater specifically to CKD diets (see Resources, page 142).

Choose prepped ingredients at the grocery store. Choosing prewashed and chopped vegetables and fruits can be a big time-saver in the kitchen, and having these items easily available may encourage your loved one to eat more vegetables and fruits. Shop for prepped ingredients like minced garlic or ginger, canned beans (instead of dried), and low-sodium sauces or frozen entrées to save time when cooking meals.

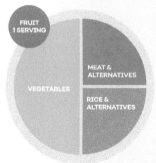

Have staple items in your pantry. Keep your pantry stocked with supplies for meals that are easy to put together when you need a break from more involved cooking. For example, with a can of tuna, you can prepare sandwiches or salad. Aim to follow the "plate method" guidelines (one-half plate vegetables, one-quarter plate protein, and one-quarter plate carbohydrates) even for meals you don't feel like cooking.

Meal Planning for Two

One of the best ways to support your loved one and help delay the progression of CKD is through nutrition. To ensure you have nutritious meals available, use the meal plan and shopping lists in chapter 2 (page 21). As your knowledge of a kidney-friendly diet grows, you will become more confident following the plate method.

You can use the plate method to plan meals that meet your loved one's protein, sodium, potassium, and phosphorus needs. Each of the recipes in this book has been carefully developed to be low in sodium. Everyone's potassium, phosphorus, and protein needs are different; it is important to look at the nutrition information provided for each recipe to determine if it fits into your loved one's kidney-friendly diet. When planning meals, choose low-potassium or low-phosphorus foods if necessary, and remember to limit protein portions if appropriate for your loved one's stage of CKD. Here are some strategies for meal planning for two.

Pick out several meals that use similar ingredients. Choose dishes that use similar ingredients so you can purchase and prepare the ingredients for a few meals at one time. If you are having similar vegetables for a few meals, wash and chop all the vegetables at the same time.

Eat the same things, mostly. Prepare meals for your loved one and customize your plate. It is okay to eat different things (for example, you may include bananas in your own oatmeal, but add a different fruit, like berries, to your loved one's bowl if they are on a potassium restriction). Meals for stages 1 to 4 will be lower in protein, and depending on your own nutrition needs, you may need to add additional protein to your portions.

Keep things flexible. If a recipe calls for a vegetable your loved one doesn't like, look for vegetables that have similar nutritional profiles to substitute. The food lists on page 122 are a great resource for learning the nutritional content of common foods. Feel free to swap in different fruits, vegetables, or proteins in meals to better suit their prefer-ences. If you want to add a salad as a side item or fruit as a dessert, go for it.

It's okay to repeat meals. Having the same thing for breakfast or any meal each day is okay if it is a balanced meal. We are creatures of habit, so follow the plate method for meals to help meet your loved one's nutritional needs, even if you're serving the same thing each day.

Choose meals with leftovers. Save time when meal planning by picking recipes that will give you leftovers for lunch the next day or another meal later in the week. Or freeze extra portions to serve later.

Caring for You, Too

As a caregiver, taking care of yourself is important, too, and it helps you support the people you love. Here are some self-care strategies.

Develop healthy ways to cope with stress. We all experience stress, so set time aside to relax and use relaxation techniques such as deep breathing, meditation, yoga, or tai chi. Seek out further support from a mental healthcare provider, if needed.

Talk to people. Join a CKD caregiver support group to meet others who understand the unique challenges of this role. Talking with others can help you feel less stressed and provide you with comfort as well as more knowledge (see Resources, page 142).

Do something for yourself. Eat a healthy diet to keep your body strong. Stay active so you have more energy. Make sure you get enough sleep. Set time aside each day to do something you enjoy, like reading, listening to music, or visiting friends.

Encourage your loved one's independence, too. Empower your loved one to be independent. This helps keep them active. It is also great for your relationship and can help prevent caregiver burnout.

Avoid the guilt. Adjusting to a new lifestyle can be difficult. When making nutrition changes, instead of feeling guilty for eating or serving foods that are not recommended, serve those foods less frequently and in smaller portions. All foods should fit when we think of a kidney-friendly diet; we just need to remember portion size. Tracking your loved one's food using tools like Cronometer or MyFitnessPal can be helpful if you need additional support with the transition.

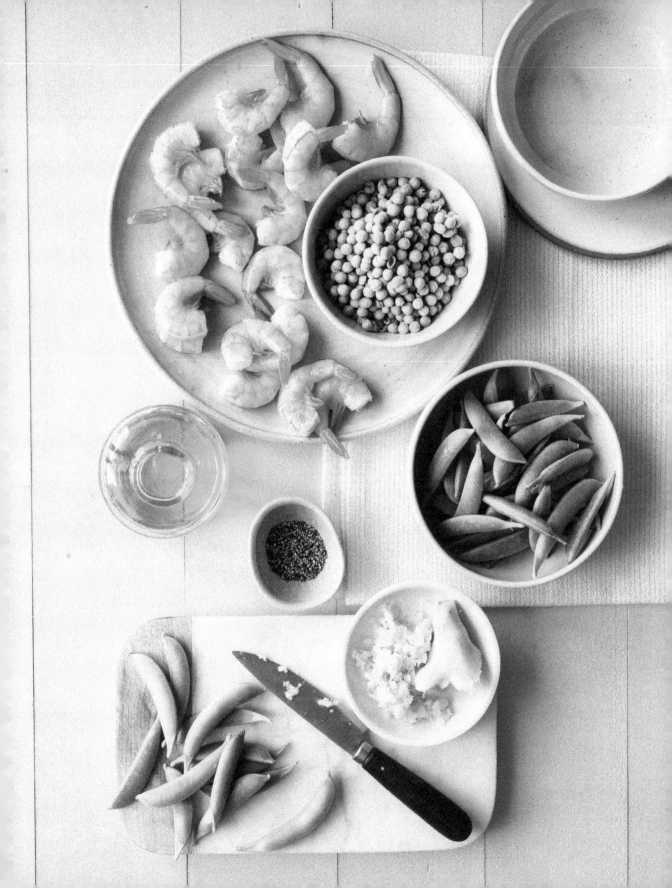

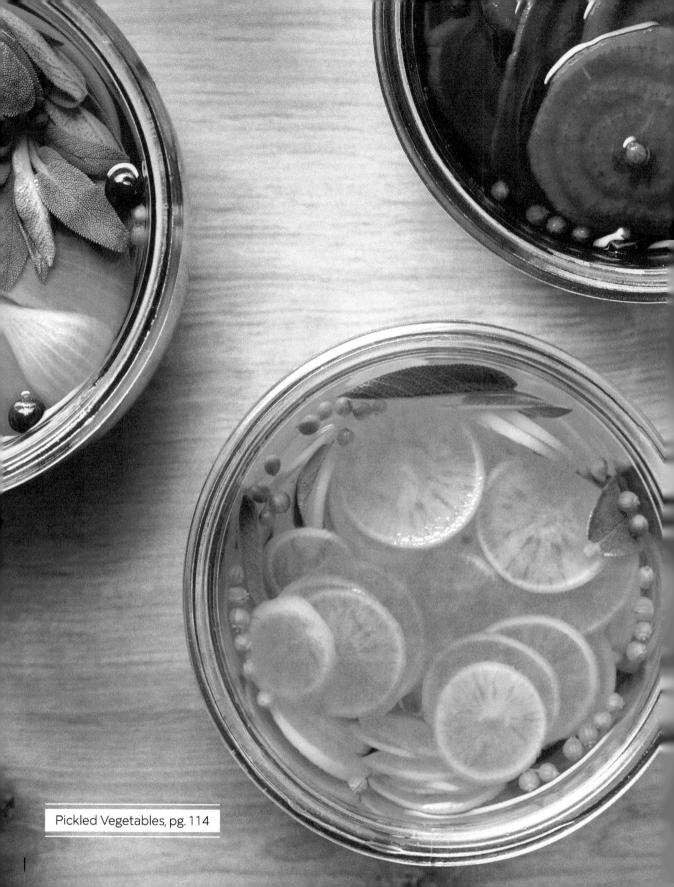

Pickled Vegetables, pg. 114

CHAPTER TWO

Stage-by-Stage Meal Plans

In this chapter, we'll review planning nutritious and delicious meals to help manage your loved one's CKD. Planning meals helps save you time and frustration in the kitchen, helps keep food costs down, and streamlines your grocery shopping.

About the Plans

Each weekly meal plan is organized by kidney disease stage, with accompanying recipes, shopping lists, and time-saving tips. At meals, remember to follow the plate method and aim for one-half plate vegetables/fruits, one-quarter plate carbohydrates, and one-quarter plate protein. Everyone has different preferences, so feel free to swap in different fruits, vegetables, carbohydrates, or proteins in meals to better suit your needs; just remember that if you make any alterations, the nutritional information will change. Everyone's nutrition needs vary, so working with a registered dietitian can help you determine the best personalized meal plan for your loved one.

These kidney-friendly meal plans are designed for two people and include three meals and two snacks. If you have more than two people in your household or want to batch cook extra portions for freezing, you can certainly do that. Batch cooking (where you make a larger batch of a recipe and freeze the excess to eat later) can be a great time-saver for meal planning. By preparing extra food ahead of time and freezing it, there will always be nutritious meals on hand for days when you have time constraints.

These meal plans include meals that can be eaten the next day or frozen for later use, so having storage containers on hand is important. Choose airtight containers with tight-fitting lids made from materials that freeze and wash well.

STAGES 1–3

	BREAKFAST	LUNCH	DINNER	SNACK	SNACK
MON.	Apple-Cinnamon Breakfast Cookies	Lemon Orzo Black Bean Salad	Chile-Lime Salmon Bowls	½ cup pineapple and 1 ounce unsalted almonds	2 cups unsalted popcorn
TUE.	Peaches and Cream Smoothie	*Leftover* Lemon Orzo Black Bean Salad	*Leftover* Chile-Lime Salmon Bowls	1 clementine and 1 ounce unsalted almonds	*Leftover* Apple-Cinnamon Breakfast Cookies
WED.	Lemon-Blueberry Oatmeal	Cauliflower and Lentil Soup	Red Wine Vinegar Baked Chicken Breast	4 ounces low-fat plain yogurt and ½ cup strawberries	½ cup celery and carrots
THU.	*Leftover* Lemon-Blueberry Oatmeal	Tuna Avocado Wrap	Turkey Kofta with Tahini	1 small apple and 1 ounce unsalted almonds	2 cup unsalted popcorn
FRI.	*Leftover* Apple-Cinnamon Breakfast Cookies	*Leftover* Tuna Avocado Wrap	*Leftover* Turkey Kofta with Tahini	4 ounces low-fat plain yogurt and ½ cup blueberries	½ cup cucumber
SAT.	Broccoli and Cheddar Mini Quiches	Pizza Bianca	Lemon-Garlic Cod	½ cup grapes and 1 ounce low-fat, low-sodium mozzarella	2 cup unsalted popcorn
SUN.	Baked French Toast	*Leftover* Pizza Bianca	*Leftover* Lemon-Garlic Cod	1 small plum and 1 ounce low-fat, low-sodium mozzarella	*Leftover* Apple-Cinnamon Breakfast Cookies

Shopping List

PRODUCE

- Apples (1 large, 1 small)
- Arugula (2 cups)
- Avocado (1 small)
- Bell pepper, orange (1 medium)
- Bell pepper, yellow (1 small)
- Blueberries, fresh (½ cup)
- Blueberries, fresh or frozen (2 cups)
- Broccoli (2 medium heads)
- Carrots (8 large)
- Cauliflower (3 medium heads)
- Celery (2 large stalks)
- Clementine (1 small)
- Cucumber (1 medium)
- Garlic, fresh (2 heads)
- Green beans (2 cups)
- Grapes (½ cup)
- Lemons (5 or 6)
- Lettuce, leaf (1 medium head)
- Lime (1)
- Radishes (4 small)
- Raspberries, fresh or frozen (1 cup)
- Onion, red (1 small)
- Onions, white (2 medium)
- Peaches, fresh or frozen (2 cups sliced)
- Pineapple, fresh (½ cup chopped)
- Plum (1 small)
- Shallots (2 medium)
- Strawberries, fresh (1½ cups)
- Tomatoes, cherry (1½ cups)

DAIRY AND EGGS

- Almond milk, plain, unsweetened (2 quarts)
- Butter, unsalted (2 sticks/8 ounces)
- Cheese, aged sharp Cheddar
- Cheese, mozzarella, low-fat, low-sodium
- Cheese, mozzarella, shredded
- Eggs (8 large)
- Yogurt, Greek, plain, low-fat (12 ounces)
- Yogurt, probiotic, vanilla, low-fat (8 ounces)

MEAT AND SEAFOOD

- Chicken breast, boneless, skinless (8 ounces)
- Cod fillets, skinless (8 ounces)
- Salmon fillets, skinless (8 ounces)
- Tuna, albacore, low-sodium (two 5-ounce cans)
- Turkey, ground, 93% lean (10 ounces)

PANTRY

- Almonds, unsalted
- Black beans, canned, no-added-salt
- Chia seeds
- Cinnamon
- Cumin
- Flour, all-purpose
- Garlic powder
- Honey
- Lentils, brown, canned, no-added-salt
- Nonstick cooking spray
- Oats, rolled (old-fashioned)
- Olive oil
- Onion powder
- Oregano, dried
- Orzo
- Paprika
- Peppercorns, black, to grind fresh as needed
- Popcorn, unsalted
- Salt
- Soy sauce, low-sodium
- Sugar
- Red pepper flakes
- Rice, parboiled
- Tahini
- Tomato paste
- Vanilla extract
- Vegetable broth, no-added-salt
- Vinegar, apple cider
- Vinegar, red wine
- Yeast, instant

OTHER

- Corn tortillas, low-sodium (four 6-inch)
- French bread (one 8-inch loaf)
- Pita breads (two 8-inch)

Prep Ahead

◆ The shopping list and recipes will provide servings for multiple days. Keep four servings available for the meal plan and freeze leftovers of the Cauliflower and Lentil Soup (page 55), Broccoli and Cheddar Mini Quiches (page 41), and Red Wine Vinegar Baked Chicken Breast (page 89).

◆ To freeze the Cauliflower and Lentil Soup, let it cool, then pour it into a zip-top freezer bag so you can lay it flat in the freezer to save space.

◆ Prepare the Broccoli and Cheddar Mini Quiches for freezing by placing them in a single layer on a piece of parchment paper in a freezer-safe container, then cover with another piece of parchment and the container lid.

◆ Prepare a double batch of Apple-Cinnamon Breakfast Cookies (page 36) and freeze extra portions. Freeze the cookies in a single layer on parchment paper in a zip-top freezer bag. Squeeze out any extra air and place flat in freezer. Take them out to thaw the day before you want to eat them. This helps keep them fresh longer.

◆ Prepare the dough for Pizza Bianca (page 58) the night before to save time.

◆ Wash and prep vegetables and fruits ahead of time for snacks for the entire week.

STAGE 4

	BREAKFAST	LUNCH	DINNER	SNACK	SNACK
MON.	Lemon-Raspberry Chia Seed Pudding	Spicy Tuna Bowls	Chicken Meatballs with Tahini	½ cup pineapple and 1 ounce unsalted almonds	Apple-Cinnamon Breakfast Cookies
TUE.	*Leftover* Lemon-Raspberry Chia Seed Pudding	*Leftover* Spicy Tuna Bowls	*Leftover* Chicken Meatballs with Tahini	1 small plum and 1 ounce low-fat, low-sodium mozzarella	½ cup cucumber
WED.	Raspberry-Vanilla Smoothie	Coleslaw Orzo Salad	Lemon-Pepper Salmon	4 ounces low-fat plain yogurt and ½ cup strawberries	*Leftover* Apple-Cinnamon Breakfast Cookies
THU.	*Leftover* Raspberry-Vanilla Smoothie	*Leftover* Coleslaw Orzo Salad	*Leftover* Lemon-Pepper Salmon	1 small apple and 1 ounce unsalted almonds	½ cup celery and carrots
FRI.	*Leftover* Apple-Cinnamon Breakfast Cookies	Herb-Marinated Tofu Sandwich	Sweet Chili Chicken	4 ounces low-fat plain yogurt and ½ cup blueberries	2 cup unsalted popcorn
SAT.	Breakfast Pizza	*Leftover* Herb- Marinated Tofu Sandwich*	*Leftover* Sweet Chili Chicken	½ cup grapes and 1 ounce low-fat, low-sodium mozzarella	½ cup cucumber
SUN.	Easy Huevos Rancheros	Greek Chickpea Power Bowl	Meatloaf Muffins with BBQ Sauce	1 clementine and 1 ounce unsalted almonds	2 cup unsalted popcorn

* Use tofu cooked the day before, but assemble the sandwich components fresh on the day you plan to serve it.

Shopping List

PRODUCE

- Apples (1 large, 1 small)
- Avocados (3 small)
- Arugula (3 cups)
- Bell pepper, green (1 medium)
- Bell pepper, orange (1 small)
- Bell pepper, red (1 small)
- Blueberries, fresh (½ cup)
- Broccoli (1 small head)
- Cabbage, green (1 small head)
- Cabbage, red (1 small head)
- Carrots (8 large)
- Cauliflower (1 small head)
- Celery (3 medium stalks)
- Clementine (1 small)
- Cucumber (4 large)
- Garlic, fresh (1 head)
- Ginger, fresh (1-inch knob)
- Grapes (½ cup)
- Green beans (3 cups)
- Kale, fresh (1 bunch)
- Lettuce, leaf (1 small head)
- Lemons (6 or 7)
- Limes (2)
- Radishes (4 small)
- Raspberries, fresh or frozen (3½ cups)
- Onion, red (1 medium)
- Onions, white (2 small)
- Pineapple, fresh (½ cup chopped)
- Plum (1 small)
- Scallions (1 small bunch)
- Serrano chile, fresh (1 small)
- Strawberries, fresh (½ cup)
- Tomatoes (2 medium)
- Tomatoes, cherry (2 cups)

DAIRY AND EGGS

- Almond milk, plain, unsweetened (about 2½ cups)
- Butter, unsalted (1 stick/4 ounces)
- Eggs, large (1 dozen)
- Cheese, mozzarella, low-fat, low-sodium
- Cheese, mozzarella, shredded
- Tofu, extra-firm (8 ounces)
- Yogurt, Greek, plain, low-fat (10 ounces)
- Yogurt, plain, low-fat (8 ounces)
- Yogurt, probiotic, plain, low-fat (8 ounces)

MEAT AND SEAFOOD

- Beef, ground, 93% lean (8 ounces)
- Chicken thighs, boneless, skinless (5 ounces)
- Chicken, ground (5 ounces)
- Salmon fillets, skinless (8 ounces)
- Tuna, skipjack, low-sodium (two 5-ounce cans)

PANTRY

- Almonds, unsalted
- Black beans, canned, no-added-salt
- Chia seeds
- Chickpeas, canned, no-added-salt
- Cinnamon
- Cornstarch
- Cumin
- Dill, dried
- Flour, all-purpose
- Garlic powder
- Nonstick cooking spray
- Oats, rolled (old-fashioned)
- Olive oil
- Onion powder
- Oregano, dried
- Orzo
- Paprika
- Peppercorns, black, to grind fresh as needed
- Red pepper flakes
- Rice, parboiled
- Salt
- Soy sauce, low-sodium
- Sugar
- Tahini
- Tomato sauce, low-sodium
- Vanilla extract
- Vinegar, apple cider
- Vinegar, red wine
- Yeast, instant

OTHER

- Corn tortillas, low-sodium (four 6-inch)
- Popcorn, unsalted
- Sourdough bread (8 slices)

Prep Ahead

- The shopping list and recipes will provide servings for multiple days. Keep four servings available for the meal plan and freeze leftovers of the Meatloaf Muffins with BBQ Sauce (page 94), Breakfast Pizza (page 44), Easy Huevos Rancheros (page 43), and Greek Chickpea Power Bowl (page 60).

- Prepare Meatloaf Muffins with BBQ Sauce for freezing by placing them in a single layer on a piece of parchment paper in a freezer-safe container, then cover with a second piece of parchment and the container lid.

- Prepare the dough for Breakfast Pizza the night before to save time.

- Breakfast Pizza can be frozen by wrapping individual slices in plastic wrap and placing them in a zip-top bag or airtight container. Easy Huevos Rancheros can be wrapped in plastic wrap and frozen in a zip-top bag. Individual portions of the Greek Chickpea Power Bowl can be frozen in airtight containers.

- Wash and prep vegetables and fruits ahead of time for snacks for the entire week.

STAGE 5

	BREAKFAST	LUNCH	DINNER	SNACK	SNACK
MON.	Peanut Butter Overnight Oats	Tzatziki Egg Salad Sandwich	Honey-Garlic Shrimp	½ cup pineapple and 1 ounce unsalted almonds	½ cup celery and carrots
TUE.	*Leftover* Peanut Butter Overnight Oats	*Leftover* Tzatziki Egg Salad Sandwich	*Leftover* Honey-Garlic Shrimp	½ cup grapes 1 ounce unsalted almonds	2 cup unsalted popcorn
WED.	Mixed Berry Protein Smoothie	Lemon-Dill Chickpea Salad Sandwich	Beef Kofta	4 ounces low-fat plain yogurt and ½ cup pineapple	Apple-Cinnamon Breakfast Cookies
THU.	*Leftover* Mixed Berry Protein Smoothie	*Leftover* Lemon-Dill Chickpea Salad Sandwich	*Leftover* Beef Kofta	1 small apple and 1 ounce unsalted almonds	2 cup unsalted popcorn
FRI.	*Leftover* Apple-Cinnamon Breakfast Cookies and 2 ounces unsalted almonds	Turkey Cobb Salad	Sheet Pan Cod with Roasted Bell Pepper and Broccolini	4 ounces low-fat plain yogurt and ½ cup pineapple	½ cup celery and carrots
SAT.	High-Protein Shakshuka with Tahini Sauce	*Leftover* Turkey Cobb Salad*	*Leftover* Sheet Pan Cod with Roasted Bell Pepper and Broccolini	1½ cup grapes and 1 ounce low-fat, low-sodium mozzarella	2 cup unsalted popcorn
SUN.	*Leftover* High-Protein Shakshuka with Tahini Sauce	Chickpea Noodle Soup	Pineapple BBQ Meatballs	1 small apple and 1 ounce low-fat, low-sodium mozzarella	½ cup celery and carrots

* Use turkey and eggs cooked the day before, but assemble the salad components fresh on the day you plan to serve it.

Shopping List

PRODUCE

- Apples (1 large, 2 small)
- Avocado (1 small)
- Banana (1 medium, 1 small)
- Bell peppers, orange (2 medium)
- Bell pepper, red (1 small)
- Bell peppers, yellow (2 medium)
- Blueberries, fresh or frozen (1 cup)
- Broccolini (1 small bunch)
- Carrots (5 large)
- Celery (4 large stalks)
- Cucumber (2 medium)
- Garlic, fresh (1 head)
- Ginger, fresh (1-inch knob)
- Grapes (1 cup)
- Green beans (2 cups)
- Herbs, fresh (optional)
- Lemons (5 medium)
- Lettuce, leaf (1 large head)
- Onions, white (2 small, 1 medium)
- Pineapple, fresh (¾ cup chopped)
- Raspberries, fresh or frozen (1 cup)
- Scallions (1 small bunch)
- Strawberries, fresh or frozen (1 cup)
- Tomatoes (4 medium)
- Tomato, cherry (2 cups)

DAIRY AND EGGS

- Almond milk, plain, unsweetened (about 3 cups)
- Butter, unsalted (1 stick/4 ounces)
- Cheese, mozzarella, low-fat, low-sodium
- Eggs, large (1½ dozen)
- Yogurt, Greek, plain, low-fat (20 ounces)
- Yogurt, plain, low-fat (8 ounces)

MEAT AND SEAFOOD

- Beef, ground, 93% lean (1½ pounds)
- Cod fillets, skinless (12 ounces)
- Shrimp, raw, peeled and deveined (1 pound)
- Turkey, breast cutlets (8 ounces)

PANTRY

- Almonds, unsalted
- Chia seeds
- Chickpeas, canned, no-added-salt
- Cinnamon
- Cumin
- Dill, dried
- Flour, all-purpose
- Garlic powder
- Honey
- Peanut butter
- Oats, rolled (old-fashioned)
- Olive oil
- Onion powder
- Oregano
- Orzo
- Paprika
- Peppercorns, black, to grind fresh as needed
- Red pepper flakes
- Salt
- Soy sauce, low-sodium
- Sugar
- Tahini
- Tomato sauce, low-sodium
- Vanilla extract
- Vegetable broth, no-added-salt
- Vinegar, apple cider
- Vinegar, red wine

OTHER

- Sourdough bread (20 slices)
- Pineapple tidbits, canned (8 ounces)
- Popcorn, unsalted

Prep Ahead

- Keep four servings available for the meal plan and freeze leftovers of the Chickpea Noodle Soup (page 65).

- Let the Chickpea Noodle Soup cool, then portion it into individual airtight containers or zip-top bags and freeze.

- Wash and prep vegetables and fruits ahead of time for snacks for the entire week.

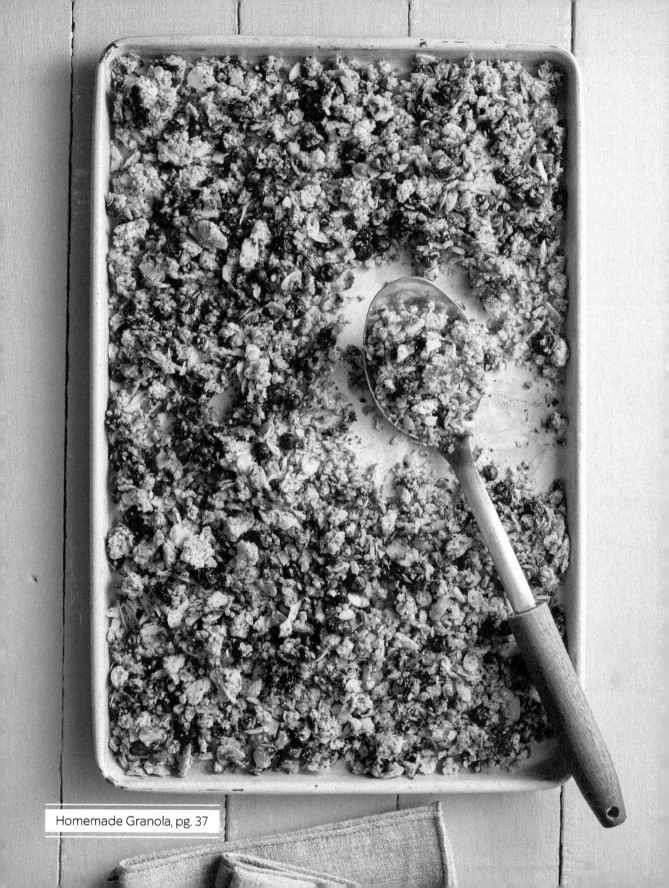

Homemade Granola, pg. 37

CHAPTER THREE

Breakfasts and Smoothies

Apple-Cinnamon Breakfast Cookies

ALL STAGES

Makes 12 cookies / Prep time: 5 minutes / **Cook time:** 10 minutes

Who wouldn't want to eat a cookie for breakfast? The addition of oats provides fiber, making these cookies extra satisfying.

1 cup rolled (old-fashioned) oats

¾ cup all-purpose flour

2 teaspoons ground cinnamon

1½ tablespoons unsalted butter, melted slightly

1 large egg

2 teaspoons vanilla extract

¼ cup unsweetened plain almond milk

1 large apple, peeled, cored, and finely chopped

1. Preheat the oven to 325°F. Line a baking sheet with parchment paper.

2. In a medium bowl, whisk together the oats, flour, and cinnamon.

3. In a small bowl, whisk together the butter, egg, vanilla, and milk. Add the wet mixture to the dry mixture and mix until incorporated. Fold in the apple pieces.

4. Drop 12 rounded scoops of the cookie dough onto the prepared baking sheet and flatten each. Bake for 10 minutes, or until the cookies are golden on the edges.

5. Let the cookies cool on the baking sheet for about 2 minutes, then transfer to a wire rack to cool completely.

TIP: The best apples for baking are those that keep their structure and have lots of flavor, such as Granny Smith, Honeycrisp, and Pink Lady.

Per serving (2 cookies): Calories: 185; Protein: 6g; Total Fat: 5g; Saturated Fat: 2g; Total Carbohydrates: 28g; Fiber: 3g; Cholesterol: 39mg; Phosphorus: 125mg; Potassium: 150mg; Sodium: 17mg; Sugar: 4g

Homemade Granola

STAGES 1–3

Makes 5 cups / Prep time: 15 minutes **/ Cook time:** 20 minutes

Granola is the perfect snack or breakfast—just add milk or yogurt and fruit for a balanced meal. Oats, the basis of granola, have many health benefits, including improving blood pressure and reducing cholesterol, making it perfect for a kidney-friendly diet. Once you've made granola from scratch, you won't go back to store-bought.

½ cup olive oil

½ cup honey

1 teaspoon vanilla extract

1 teaspoon ground cinnamon

3 cups rolled (old-fashioned) oats

½ cup sliced almonds

¼ cup chia seeds

½ cup dried cranberries

1. Preheat the oven to 300°F. Line a baking sheet with parchment paper.

2. In a large bowl, whisk together the oil, honey, vanilla, and cinnamon. Add the oats, almonds, and chia seeds and stir to coat well.

3. Spread the mixture evenly on the prepared baking sheet and press it down. Bake for 20 minutes, or until golden brown, stirring once halfway through.

4. Let the granola cool, then break it into pieces, add the dried cranberries, and mix well.

TIP: Store the granola in an airtight container at room temperature for up to 2 weeks or freeze for longer storage.

Per serving (½ cup): Calories: 336; Protein: 7g; Total Fat: 17g; Saturated Fat: 2g; Total Carbohydrates: 42g; Fiber: 6g; Cholesterol: 0mg; Phosphorus: 226mg; Potassium: 196mg; Sodium: 3mg; Sugar: 18g

Lemon-Blueberry Oatmeal

STAGES 1–3

Serves 4 / Prep time: 5 minutes / **Cook time:** 10 minutes

This easy oatmeal contains bluberries, a low-glycemic-index berry (see Tip), food that helps control blood glucose levels for those who have diabetes.

4 cups unsweetened plain almond milk

2 cups rolled (old-fashioned) oats

1 tablespoon honey

¼ cup chia seeds

4 teaspoons grated lemon zest

Juice of 1 lemon

2 cups fresh or frozen blueberries

1. In a medium saucepan, bring the milk to a slight simmer over medium heat, then add the oats, honey, chia seeds, and lemon zest. Bring the mixture to a boil, then reduce the heat to low and simmer for 5 minutes, stirring occasionally. Remove from the heat.

2. Stir in the lemon juice and top with the blueberries before serving.

TIP: The glycemic index is a measure of how quickly foods cause blood glucose levels to rise. Some great low-glycemic-index fruits include apples, berries, peaches, pears, pomegranates, and plums.

Per serving (1½ cups): Calories: 351; Protein: 12g; Total Fat: 11g; Saturated Fat: 1g; Total Carbohydrates: 55g; Fiber: 12g; Cholesterol: 0mg; Phosphorus: 409mg; Potassium: 427mg; Sodium: 129mg; Sugar: 12g

Peaches and Cream Smoothie

STAGES 1–3

Serves 4 / Prep time: 5 minutes

This smoothie gets its creamy texture from probiotic yogurt. Probiotic yogurts have added beneficial bacteria and can help regulate the digestive tract. Bonus: This smoothie is a great on-the-go breakfast for hectic mornings.

1 cup vanilla probiotic yogurt

2 cups fresh or frozen peach slices

1½ cups unsweetened plain almond milk

1 teaspoon vanilla extract

½ cup ice

1. Combine the yogurt, peaches, milk, vanilla, and ice in a blender and blend until smooth.

2. Pour into glasses and serve immediately.

TIP: Leftover portions of this smoothie can be frozen and enjoyed later. Or freeze in ice pop molds for a great dessert on a hot day.

Per serving (1 cup): Calories: 80; Protein: 3g; Total Fat: 3g; Saturated Fat: 1g; Total Carbohydrates: 10g; Fiber: 1g; Cholesterol: 8mg; Phosphorus: 80mg; Potassium: 293mg; Sodium: 69mg; Sugar: 9g

Baked French Toast

STAGES 1–3

Serves 4 / Prep time: 10 minutes / **Cook time:** 25 minutes

French toast originated in medieval times as a way to use up day-old or slightly stale bread. The bread soaks up the egg custard, now traditionally made with cinnamon and vanilla, to make a decadently delicious brunch meal.

Nonstick cooking spray

3 large eggs

¾ cup unsweetened plain almond milk

2 teaspoons ground cinnamon

½ teaspoon vanilla extract

8 (1-inch-thick) French bread slices

1 cup fresh or frozen raspberries

1 cup fresh or frozen blueberries

1 cup fresh strawberries, halved

1. Preheat the oven to 400°F. Coat a 9-inch square baking dish with nonstick spray.

2. In a large bowl, combine the eggs, milk, cinnamon, and vanilla. Submerge the bread in the egg mixture and let it soak for 2 minutes to absorb the custard.

3. Place the bread in the prepared baking dish. Bake for 15 minutes, then remove the baking dish from the oven and carefully turn the bread over. Bake for 10 minutes more, or until the bread is golden brown on both sides.

4. In a small bowl, mix the berries together. Top each slice of French toast with the mixed berries before serving.

TIP: For a denser result, use slightly stale French bread for this recipe. You can also use regular sliced bread.

Per serving (2 slices French toast and ¾ cup berries): Calories: 457; Protein: 19g; Total Fat: 7g; Saturated Fat: 2g; Total Carbohydrates: 80g; Fiber: 7g; Cholesterol: 140mg; Phosphorus: 233mg; Potassium: 346mg; Sodium: 325mg; Sugar: 13g

Broccoli and Cheddar Mini Quiches

STAGES 1–3

Makes 12 mini quiches / Prep time: 15 minutes / **Cook time:** 35 minutes

Easier and quicker than the full-size version, these mini quiches are perfect for a filling weekday breakfast. You can even prepare them ahead of time, because they are easy to freeze and reheat. Best of all, you can customize the ingredients to your liking.

Nonstick cooking spray

All-purpose flour, for dusting

Pie Crust (page 119)

4 large eggs

½ cup unsweetened plain almond milk

1 teaspoon freshly ground black pepper

½ teaspoon red pepper flakes

½ cup chopped white onion

½ cup chopped broccoli florets

½ cup shredded aged sharp Cheddar cheese

1. Preheat the oven to 375°F. Coat a muffin tin with nonstick spray.

2. On a lightly floured counter, using your hands or a rolling pin, flatten each dough ball into a round. With a small cookie cutter or the rim of a glass, cut out 12 rounds of dough.

3. Place one round of dough in each well of the prepared muffin tin and bake for 10 minutes.

4. Meanwhile, in a medium bowl, whisk the eggs and milk until light and airy. Add the black pepper, red pepper flakes, onion, broccoli, and cheese and stir to combine.

5. Remove the muffin tin from the oven. Divide the egg mixture evenly among the quiche crusts and bake for 15 to 25 minutes, until the eggs are set.

Per serving (2 mini quiches): Calories: 439; Protein: 11g; Total Fat: 17g; Saturated Fat: 16g; Total Carbohydrates: 37g; Fiber: 2g; Cholesterol: 188mg; Phosphorus: 173mg; Potassium: 161mg; Sodium: 127mg; Sugar: 3g

Veggie Egg Bake

STAGES 1–3

Serves 4 / Prep time: 10 minutes / **Cook time:** 20 minutes

This egg bake is super convenient for busy mornings or entertaining on the weekend. Eggs are incredibly nutritious and full of vitamins and minerals, as well as a great source of inexpensive protein.

Nonstick cooking spray

4 large eggs

3 tablespoons unsweetened plain almond milk

1 teaspoon minced garlic

1 teaspoon freshly ground black pepper

1 cup diced red bell pepper

1 cup arugula

½ cup diced white onion

½ cup shredded Cheddar cheese

2 sourdough bread slices, cut into cubes

1. Preheat the oven to 350°F. Coat an 8-inch square baking dish with nonstick spray.

2. In a medium bowl, whisk together the eggs, milk, garlic, and black pepper. Add the bell pepper, arugula, onion, cheese, and bread and mix well.

3. Pour the mixture into the prepared baking dish. Bake for 20 minutes, or until the eggs are set.

TIP: Substitute low-sodium feta or sharp Swiss cheese for the Cheddar to change the flavor profile.

Per serving (1 cup): Calories: 338; Protein: 18g; Total Fat: 11g; Saturated Fat: 5g; Total Carbohydrates: 40g; Fiber: 2g; Cholesterol: 200mg; Phosphorus: 254mg; Potassium: 257mg; Sodium: 467mg; Sugar: 6g

Easy Huevos Rancheros

STAGES 1–4

Serves 4 / Prep time: 5 minutes **/ Cook time:** 10 minutes

Huevos rancheros is Spanish for "rancher's eggs," and this simple-to-prepare version is sure to spice up your morning. It includes a fried egg served with black beans and avocado on top of a corn tortilla, in perfect portions for a kidney-friendly diet.

1 tablespoon olive oil

4 (6-inch) low-sodium corn tortillas

4 large eggs

1 (15-ounce) can no-added-salt black beans, drained and rinsed

¼ cup lime juice

1 teaspoon red pepper flakes

2 teaspoons freshly ground black pepper

½ ripe avocado, sliced

1 medium tomato, chopped

1. In a large nonstick skillet, heat the oil over medium-high heat. Once hot, fry each tortilla, one at a time, for 1 to 2 minutes, until the edges are crisp. Transfer to four serving plates and set aside.

2. Crack the eggs into the same skillet and fry until the egg whites are opaque and the yolks have risen a bit but are still soft (or cook to your liking).

3. While the eggs are cooking, in a small bowl, combine the black beans, lime juice, red pepper flakes, and black pepper and lightly mash with a fork.

4. Spread the bean mixture evenly over each tortilla and top with the avocado, tomato, and a cooked egg.

TIP: If you have leftover bean mixture, store it in an airtight container in the refrigerator for up to 3 days. Reheat in a skillet until bubbling and warm.

Per serving (1 tortilla, 1 egg, and one-quarter bean mixture):
Calories: 299; Protein: 14g; Total Fat: 12g; Saturated Fat: 2g; Total Carbohydrates: 34g; Fiber: 9g; Cholesterol: 186mg; Phosphorus: 299mg; Potassium: 499mg; Sodium: 79mg; Sugar: 2g

Breakfast Pizza

STAGES 1–4

Serves 4 / **Prep time:** 15 minutes / **Cook time:** 15 minutes

Pizza for breakfast? Why not! This pizza recipe is a great weekend breakfast that is simple, delicious, and makes great leftovers. You can customize the toppings to use whatever you have in the refrigerator. Adding vegetables to meals helps add fiber to the plate.

Nonstick cooking spray

All-purpose flour, for dusting

Pizza Dough (page 118)

1 tablespoon olive oil

1 cup shredded mozza-
    rella cheese

1 cup chopped tomato

½ cup thinly sliced red onion

1 cup arugula

½ cup thinly sliced orange
    bell pepper

4 large eggs

1 tablespoon dried oregano

1. Preheat the oven to 450°F. Coat two large baking sheets with nonstick spray.

2. On a lightly floured counter, using your hands or a rolling pin, work each dough ball into a round. Place one round of dough on each prepared baking sheet.

3. Drizzle the dough with the olive oil and sprinkle with the mozzarella, dividing it evenly. Top each pizza evenly with the tomato, onion, arugula, and bell pepper.

4. Crack 2 eggs onto each pizza. Sprinkle the oregano on top and bake for 10 to 15 minutes, until the crust is golden brown, the egg whites are opaque, and the egg yolks have risen a bit but are still soft (or cooked to your liking).

5. Cut each pizza into four slices and serve.

TIP: For a low-cholesterol option, skip the egg yolks and use just the whites instead. Simply mix the vegetables with the egg whites in a scramble and bake on top of the dough.

Per serving (2 slices): Calories: 325; Protein: 17g; Total Fat: 15g; Saturated Fat: 6g; Total Carbohydrates: 29g; Fiber: 2g; Cholesterol: 208mg; Phosphorus: 257mg; Potassium: 308mg; Sodium: 492mg; Sugar: 3g

Lemon-Raspberry Chia Seed Pudding

STAGE 4

Serves 4 / Prep time: 5 minutes / **Chill Time:** 15 minutes

Chia seeds are a great source of fiber and omega-3 fatty acids. When chia seeds are mixed with almond milk, they make a sort of pudding that takes on the flavor of the added fruit. This tangy-and-tart breakfast will get you and your taste buds moving for the day.

½ cup chia seeds

2 cups unsweetened plain almond milk

1 teaspoon vanilla extract

1 tablespoon lemon juice

2 cups fresh or frozen raspberries

1. In a small bowl, stir together the chia seeds, milk, vanilla, and lemon juice.

2. Cover and refrigerate the mixture for at least 15 minutes or up to overnight. The pudding is ready when it has a thick and creamy texture.

3. Top with the raspberries before serving.

TIP: Chia seeds are a great topper on salads and roasted vegetables. As a source of fiber and antioxidants, they are a great kidney-friendly addition to any meal.

Per serving (½ cup pudding and ½ cup raspberries): Calories: 118; Protein: 5g; Total Fat: 5g; Saturated Fat: 1g; Total Carbohydrates: 14g; Fiber: 9g; Cholesterol: 0mg; Phosphorus: 140mg; Potassium: 209mg; Sodium: 38mg; Sugar: 3g

Raspberry-Vanilla Smoothie

STAGE 4

Serves 4 / Prep time: 5 minutes

This smoothie is packed with fruits and vegetables, which makes it an easy way to sneak fiber into your diet to help keep your bowels regular. Place in individual Mason jars with lids for easy storage and a convenient grab-and-go container.

1 cup low-fat plain probiotic yogurt

1½ cups fresh or frozen raspberries

¼ cup chopped kale leaves

¼ cup cauliflower florets

2 teaspoons vanilla extract

1½ cups water

½ cup ice cubes

1. Combine the yogurt, raspberries, kale, cauliflower, vanilla, water, and ice cubes in a blender and blend until smooth.

2. Pour into glasses and serve immediately.

Per serving (1 cup): Calories: 71; Protein: 4g; Total Fat: 1g; Saturated Fat: 0g; Total Carbohydrates: 11g; Fiber: 3g; Cholesterol: 4mg; Phosphorus: 106mg; Potassium: 241mg; Sodium: 46mg; Sugar: 7g

Mixed Berry Protein Smoothie

STAGE 5

Serves 4 / Prep time: 5 minutes

This recipe is a refreshing and healthy combination of berries that are packed with antioxidants. Did you know that frozen berries are flash-chilled at their peak nutrition and ripeness? This means you can enjoy nutritious fruits all year round!

1 cup fresh or frozen blueberries

1 cup fresh or frozen raspberries

1 cup fresh or frozen strawberries

1 small banana

1 tablespoon chia seeds

1 tablespoon peanut butter

1½ cups unsweetened plain almond milk

1 cup low-fat plain Greek yogurt

8 ounces silken tofu

½ cup ice

1. Combine the blueberries, raspberries, strawberries, banana, chia seeds, peanut butter, milk, yogurt, tofu, and ice in a blender and blend until smooth.

2. Pour into glasses and serve immediately.

Per serving (2 cups): Calories: 258; Protein: 15g; Total Fat: 10g; Saturated Fat: 2g; Total Carbohydrates: 32g; Fiber: 6g; Cholesterol: 8mg; Phosphorus: 270mg; Potassium: 491mg; Sodium: 99mg; Sugar: 17g

Peanut Butter Overnight Oats

STAGE 5

Makes 4 cups / Prep time: 10 minutes

These oats are soaked overnight in milk and yogurt to give you a creamy, salty, sweet breakfast that can be prepared ahead of time. Overnight oats are a quick-and-easy breakfast option that is packed with protein and fiber.

1 cup rolled
   (old-fashioned) oats
2 cups unsweetened plain
   almond milk
1½ cups low-fat plain
   Greek yogurt
4 teaspoons ground
   cinnamon
¼ cup chia seeds
¼ cup peanut butter
1 medium banana, sliced

1. In a medium bowl, mix together the oats, milk, yogurt, cinnamon, chia seeds, and peanut butter.

2. Cover the bowl (or divide the oat mixture among four individual airtight containers) and refrigerate overnight.

3. Serve cold, or warm in the microwave for 30 seconds. Top with the banana slices just before serving.

TIP: These oats are a great snack after dialysis to help replace protein lost during treatment.

Per serving (1 cup): Calories: 302; Protein: 22g; Total Fat: 15g; Saturated Fat: 3g; Total Carbohydrates: 28g; Fiber: 8g; Cholesterol: 8mg; Phosphorus: 441mg; Potassium: 480mg; Sodium: 122mg; Sugar: 2g

High-Protein Shakshuka with Tahini Sauce

STAGE 5

Serves 4 / Prep time: 15 minutes / **Cook time:** 30 minutes

Shakshuka is a one-pot Middle Eastern dish of eggs, tomato, and rich seasoning. This recipe can be made as spicy as you wish, so try adding extra paprika or hot pepper, if you like.

½ teaspoon ground cumin

1 teaspoon dried oregano

1 teaspoon red
   pepper flakes

1 tablespoon olive oil

1 small white onion, sliced

1 garlic clove, minced

2 medium yellow bell pep-
   pers, sliced

3 medium tomatoes,
   chopped

8 large eggs

Tahini Sauce (page 112)

4 small sourdough
   bread slices

1. Preheat the oven to 400°F.

2. In a medium ovenproof skillet or sauté pan, toast the cumin, oregano, and red pepper flakes over medium-high heat for 1 minute. Add the oil, onion, garlic, and bell peppers and cook, stirring often, for 5 minutes, or until the vegetables are soft.

3. Add the tomatoes, reduce the heat to medium, and simmer for 10 minutes, stirring once or twice.

4. Crack the eggs into the pan, distributing them as evenly as possible. Bake for 15 minutes, or until the egg whites are opaque and the yolks have risen a bit but are still soft (or cook to your liking).

5. Top with the tahini sauce and enjoy with a slice of bread.

Per serving (2 cups): Calories: 400; Protein: 21g; Total Fat: 15g; Saturated Fat: 4g; Total Carbohydrates: 46g; Fiber: 4g; Cholesterol: 372mg; Phosphorus: 319mg; Potassium: 546mg; Sodium: 503mg; Sugar: 6g

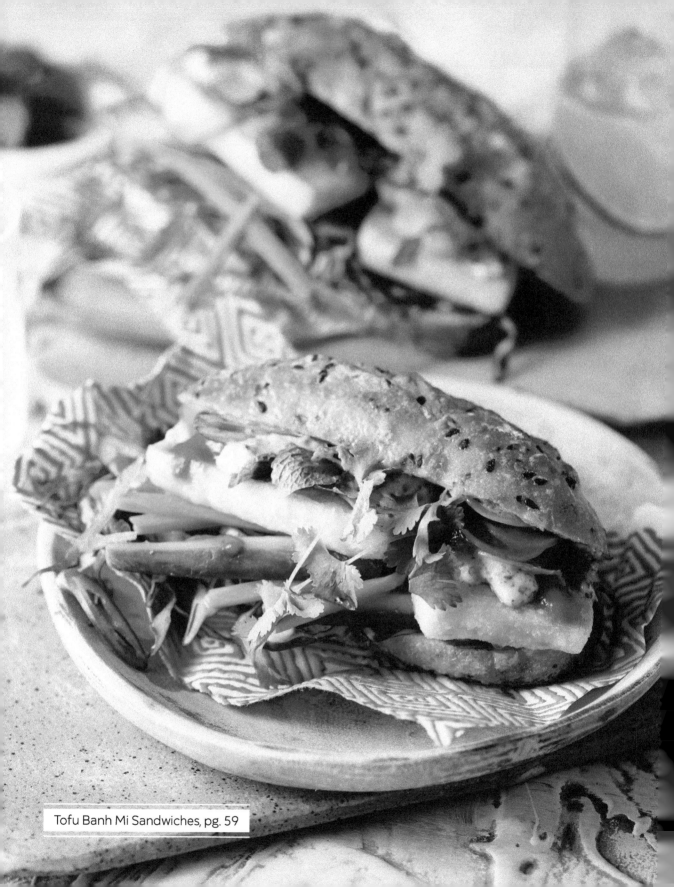

Tofu Banh Mi Sandwiches, pg. 59

CHAPTER FOUR

Vegetarian Mains

Refreshing Caprese Pasta Salad

STAGES 1–3

Serves 6 / Prep time: 5 minutes / **Cook time:** 15 minutes

A caprese salad is an Italian salad often served in the summer to make use of ripe tomatoes. This caprese includes a twist of red wine vinegar and oregano that will leave your taste buds asking for more. This dish uses orzo, but you can use any small pasta you have at home, like shells or penne.

8 ounces orzo

½ cup olive oil

¼ cup red wine vinegar

4 garlic cloves, minced

3 tablespoons
 dried oregano

1 tablespoon red
 pepper flakes

1 teaspoon freshly ground
 black pepper

1 cup cherry toma-
 toes, halved

4 ounces bocconcini (moz-
 zarella balls), quartered

1 cup arugula

1. Cook the orzo as directed on the package, drain, and set aside to cool.

2. In a medium bowl, whisk together the oil, vinegar, garlic, oregano, red pepper flakes, and black pepper.

3. Add the tomatoes, mozzarella, and arugula to the bowl and toss. Add the cooled orzo and toss to combine.

TIP: This pasta salad can be stored in an airtight container in the refrigerator for up to 2 days.

Per serving (2 cups): Calories: 368; Protein: 9g; Total Fat: 23g; Saturated Fat: 5g; Total Carbohydrates: 31g; Fiber: 2g; Cholesterol: 15mg; Phosphorus: 134mg; Potassium: 180mg; Sodium: 124mg; Sugar: 2g

Lemon Orzo Black Bean Salad

STAGES 1–3

Serves 4 / Prep time: 5 minutes **/ Cook time:** 15 minutes

This orzo and black bean salad, with its refreshing lemon dressing, is the perfect dish for a summer day. With a handful of pantry staples, this salad comes together in a snap and can be prepared ahead of time, if needed.

4 ounces orzo

¼ cup lemon juice

¼ cup olive oil

1 teaspoon dried oregano

1 teaspoon freshly ground
  black pepper

1 (15-ounce) can
  no-added-salt black
  beans, drained and rinsed

1 cup cherry tomatoes,
  halved

1. Cook the orzo as directed on the package. Reserve ½ cup of the cooking water, then drain and set aside to cool.

2. In a medium bowl, whisk together the reserved orzo cooking water, the lemon juice, oil, oregano, and pepper.

3. Add the beans, tomatoes, and cooled orzo to the bowl with the dressing and toss to combine, making sure everything is well coated.

TIP: For a well-cooked orzo salad, cook the orzo just past al dente. This helps keep it soft when it cools.

Per serving (1 cup): Calories: 320; Protein: 10g; Total Fat: 14g; Saturated Fat: 2g; Total Carbohydrates: 39g; Fiber: 7g; Cholesterol: 0mg; Phosphorus: 154mg; Potassium: 399mg; Sodium: 5mg; Sugar: 2g

Marinated Lentil Salad

STAGES 1–3

Serves 4 / Prep time: 10 minutes

Lentils are a legume, with most of the world's production coming from Canada and India. Lentils come in a variety of colors: red, yellow, green, brown, and black. Green and brown lentils tend to hold their shape and are best used in salads; red and yellow lentils disintegrate as they cook, so they are better for soups. Inexpensive and quick to prepare, lentils are a great source of fiber and plant-based protein. Serve this dish with your favorite garden salad.

2 tablespoons olive oil

2 tablespoons lemon juice

1 tablespoon red
wine vinegar

1 teaspoon freshly ground
black pepper

2 scallions, green parts
only, chopped

1 cup diced yellow
bell pepper

1 cup cherry tomatoes,
halved

1 (15-ounce) can
no-added-salt brown len-
tils, drained and rinsed

1. In a medium bowl, whisk together the oil, lemon juice, vinegar, and black pepper.

2. Add the scallions, bell pepper, tomatoes, and lentils to the bowl and toss to coat with the dressing.

TIP: This salad tastes better the longer it marinates, so it is great for leftovers.

Per serving (1 cup): Calories: 169; Protein: 8g; Total Fat: 7g; Saturated Fat: 1g; Total Carbohydrates: 20g; Fiber: 7g; Cholesterol: 0mg; Phosphorus: 156mg; Potassium: 480mg; Sodium: 6mg; Sugar: 3g

Cauliflower and Lentil Soup

STAGES 1–3

Makes 12 cups / Prep time: 10 minutes / **Cook time:** 15 minutes

This Indian-inspired dish is a filling soup that makes a budget-friendly meal. By blending the vegetables and lentils, you end up with a soup with a creamy and smooth consistency. Top it off with a dollop of yogurt and sprinkling of fresh cilantro.

1 tablespoon olive oil

4 garlic cloves, minced

1 medium white
   onion, chopped

1 cup chopped carrots

3 cups cauliflower florets

6 cups no-added-salt
   vegetable broth

2 cups water

1 (15-ounce) can
   no-added-salt brown lentils, drained and rinsed

1 teaspoon freshly ground
   black pepper

2 teaspoons lemon juice

1. In a large pot, heat the oil over medium heat. Add the garlic, onion, and carrots and cook, stirring, until the onion is translucent and soft, about 5 minutes.

2. Add the cauliflower, broth, and water and increase the heat to high. Bring to a boil, then reduce the heat to medium and simmer until the cauliflower is tender, about 6 minutes.

3. Add the lentils, pepper, and lemon juice and simmer for 3 minutes more. Remove the soup from the heat.

4. Carefully pour the soup into a blender and, holding a towel over the lid, blend until smooth (or use an immersion blender to puree the soup directly in the pot).

TIP: Kick up the flavor of this soup and give it a nutritional boost by adding 1 teaspoon ground turmeric and 1 teaspoon curry powder, both of which are powerful anti-inflammatory seasonings.

Per serving (2 cups): Calories: 110; Protein: 6g; Total Fat: 3g; Saturated Fat: 0g; Total Carbohydrates: 17g; Fiber: 6g; Cholesterol: 0mg; Phosphorus: 129mg; Potassium: 447mg; Sodium: 34mg; Sugar: 4g

Black Bean and Couscous Power Bowl

STAGES 1–3

Serves 4 / **Prep time:** 10 minutes / **Cook time:** 10 minutes

Couscous is a traditional grain-like pasta from North Africa. Made from semolina, tiny grains of couscous cook quickly and take on the flavors of other ingredients. And because couscous is low in potassium, it's a great option for those on a CKD diet.

1½ cups no-added-salt vegetable broth

1 cup couscous

2 tablespoons lemon juice

1 tablespoon olive oil

1 teaspoon freshly ground black pepper

1 tablespoon Mexican Seasoning (page 120)

1 (15-ounce) can no-added-salt black beans, drained and rinsed

2 cups arugula

1 cup cherry tomatoes, halved

½ cup diced red onion

1. In a medium pot, bring the broth to a boil over high heat. Add the couscous, cover, and remove from the heat. Let sit for 5 minutes, then fluff the couscous with a fork.

2. In a small bowl, stir together the lemon juice, oil, pepper, and Mexican seasoning.

3. Add the black beans to the pot with the couscous and stir to combine.

4. Divide the arugula among four plates and top each evenly with the tomatoes, onion, and couscous-bean mixture.

Per serving (2 cups): Calories: 294; Protein: 12g; Total Fat: 4g; Saturated Fat: 1g; Total Carbohydrates: 52g; Fiber: 9g; Cholesterol: 0mg; Phosphorus: 183mg; Potassium: 455mg; Sodium: 10mg; Sugar: 2g

Black Bean Burgers

STAGES 1–3

Serves 4 / Prep time: 10 minutes **/ Cook time:** 10 minutes

Black bean burgers are a great plant-based option for burger night, and these patties are packed with flavor, so they won't disappoint. These burgers are soft on the inside but crisp and crunchy on the outside, but most important, they come together in a snap.

1 (15-ounce) can
  no-added-salt black
  beans, drained and rinsed
2 tablespoons olive
  oil, divided
1 tablespoon lemon juice
1 tablespoon dried oregano
2 garlic cloves, minced
½ cup rolled
  (old-fashioned) oats
Tzatziki Sauce (page 113)
4 hamburger buns
8 cucumber slices
4 tomato slices

1. Combine the black beans, 1 tablespoon of the oil, the lemon juice, oregano, and garlic in a food processor and pulse 3 or 4 times, until the beans are smashed. (Alternatively, combine the ingredients in a bowl and use a potato masher to smash the beans.)

2. Add the oats and stir until well combined. Using your hands, form the mixture into four equal-size patties.

3. In a medium skillet, heat the remaining 1 tablespoon oil over medium heat. Add the patties and cook for 3 minutes per side, or until golden brown.

4. Divide the tzatziki sauce evenly among the buns, spreading it over the cut sides of the top and bottom halves of each. Top each bottom bun with a black bean patty, two cucumber slices, and a tomato slice, then finish with the bun tops.

Per serving (1 burger): Calories: 314; Protein: 12g; Total Fat: 10g; Saturated Fat: 2g; Total Carbohydrates: 46g; Fiber: 8g; Cholesterol: 0mg; Phosphorus: 203mg; Potassium: 371mg; Sodium: 212mg; Sugar: 3g

Pizza Bianca

STAGES 1–3

Serves 4 / Prep time: 15 minutes / **Cook time:** 15 minutes

Pizza bianca, or "white pizza," is pizza without tomato sauce (which is high in potassium). Instead, it is topped with olive oil and herbs. Customize it by adding your favorite low-potassium vegetables like bell pepper or onion.

Nonstick cooking spray

All-purpose flour, for dusting

Pizza Dough (page 118)

1 tablespoon olive oil

2 garlic cloves, minced

2 teaspoons dried oregano

1 cup shredded mozzarella cheese

2 teaspoons red pepper flakes

2 cups arugula

1. Preheat the oven to 450°F. Coat two large baking sheets with nonstick spray.

2. On a lightly floured counter, using your hands or a rolling pin, work each dough ball into a round. Place one round of dough on each prepared baking sheet.

3. Brush each round of dough with oil, then top evenly with the garlic and oregano. Bake for 10 minutes, or until the crust is golden and baked.

4. Remove the pizza crusts from the oven and top with the mozzarella and red pepper flakes. Bake for 3 minutes more, or until the cheese has melted.

5. Remove the pizzas from the oven, top evenly with the arugula, and cut each into four slices.

TIP: This pizza crisps up great on a baking sheet, but if you have a pizza stone, you can easily cook it on that instead.

Per serving (2 slices): Calories: 238; Protein: 11g; Total Fat: 10g; Saturated Fat: 4g; Total Carbohydrates: 26g; Fiber: 1g; Cholesterol: 22mg; Phosphorus: 144mg; Potassium: 109mg; Sodium: 326mg; Sugar: 0g

Tofu Banh Mi Sandwiches

STAGES 1–3

Serves 4 / Prep time: 20 minutes / **Cook time:** 20 minutes

Banh mi are Vietnamese street food sandwiches served on a crunchy, short baguette and topped with pickled vegetables. This recipe is a delicious plant-based alternative to a classic banh mi. Plant-based proteins are important for delaying the progression of CKD.

8 ounces extra-firm tofu

1 tablespoon olive oil

2 tablespoons low-sodium soy sauce

2 tablespoons lime juice

2 garlic cloves, minced

1 teaspoon minced fresh ginger

1 teaspoon freshly ground black pepper

¼ cup low-fat plain Greek yogurt

2 teaspoons red pepper flakes

1 teaspoon low-sodium hot sauce (optional)

4 (4-inch) baguette pieces, split lengthwise

Pickled Vegetables (page 114)

½ cup arugula (optional)

1. Slice the tofu into eight pieces and place on paper towels to drain.

2. In a small bowl, mix together the oil, soy sauce, lime juice, garlic, ginger, and black pepper. Add the tofu and toss to coat every piece. Set aside to marinate for 15 minutes.

3. Heat a medium skillet over medium heat. Place the tofu in the skillet and cook for 5 to 10 minutes, until golden brown on both sides.

4. In a small bowl, combine the yogurt, red pepper flakes, and hot sauce, if using.

5. Spread the yogurt dressing over each baguette, add two pieces of the tofu to each, and top with the pickled vegetables and arugula, if using.

TIP: This recipe can be made with chicken or pork as the protein instead of the tofu.

Per serving (1 sandwich): Calories: 154; Protein: 9g; Total Fat: 8g; Saturated Fat: 1g; Total Carbohydrates: 13g; Fiber: 1g; Cholesterol: 2mg; Phosphorus: 128mg; Potassium: 163mg; Sodium: 390mg; Sugar: 1g

Greek Chickpea Power Bowl

STAGES 1–4

Serves 4 / Prep time: 10 minutes **/ Cook time:** 20 minutes

This Greek-inspired power bowl comes together quickly for a quick, healthy, plant-based meal in a pinch. By using pantry staples and adding a pop of color with fresh vegetables, you'll want to work this into your weeknight rotation.

2 cups parboiled rice

1 (15-ounce) can no-added-salt chickpeas, drained and rinsed

1 tablespoon lemon juice

1 tablespoon olive oil

1 tablespoon dried oregano

1½ teaspoons dried dill

1 teaspoon freshly ground black pepper

2 cups diced cucumbers

2 cups cherry tomatoes, halved

2 cups arugula

Tzatziki Sauce (page 113)

1. Cook the rice as directed on the package and set aside.

2. In a large bowl, combine the chickpeas, lemon juice, oil, oregano, dill, and pepper.

3. Add the rice, cucumbers, tomatoes, and arugula to the bowl with the herbed chickpeas and mix well. Divide among four individual serving bowls and top with tzatziki.

TIP: Chickpeas are a great source of iron and fiber and easily take on the flavors of this dish, but they can be swapped out for black beans or lentils.

Per serving (2½ cups): Calories: 416; Protein: 12g; Total Fat: 6g; Saturated Fat: 1g; Total Carbohydrates: 79g; Fiber: 9g; Cholesterol: 0mg; Phosphorus: 192mg; Potassium: 492mg; Sodium: 17mg; Sugar: 6g

Coleslaw Orzo Salad

STAGE 4

Serves 4 / Prep time: 5 minutes **/ Cook time:** 15 minutes

This unique coleslaw is made with a creamy, sour dressing that is a flavorful twist on a traditional coleslaw. Cabbage is a low-potassium vegetable full of vitamins, antioxidants, and fiber. This recipe makes an easy-to-prepare main dish, but you can also serve it as a hearty side.

6 ounces orzo

2 cups shredded
green cabbage

1 cup shredded red cabbage

1 cup shredded carrots

2 scallions, green parts
only, chopped

½ cup low-fat plain
Greek yogurt

1 tablespoon sugar

1 tablespoon lemon juice

1 tablespoon red
wine vinegar

2 teaspoons freshly ground
black pepper

1. Cook the orzo as directed on the package, drain, and set aside to cool.

2. In a large bowl, combine the green and red cabbage, carrots, and scallions.

3. In a small bowl, stir together the yogurt, sugar, lemon juice, vinegar, and pepper.

4. Pour the dressing over the cabbage mixture. Add the cooled orzo and toss to combine.

5. Store leftovers in an airtight container in the refrigerator for up to 2 days.

Per serving (2 cups): Calories: 212; Protein: 7g; Total Fat: 1g; Saturated Fat: 1g; Total Carbohydrates: 44g; Fiber: 4g; Cholesterol: 4mg; Phosphorus: 82mg; Potassium: 284mg; Sodium: 46mg; Sugar: 1g

Herb-Marinated Tofu Sandwich

STAGE 4

Makes 4 sandwiches / Prep time: 20 minutes (or up to 8 hours marinating) /
Cook time: 20 minutes

The tofu for these sandwiches is perfectly marinated with herbs and citrus juice and pan-seared until crispy on the outside. This dish is a great plant-based lunch. If potassium is not a concern, try adding more avocado slices for an extra creamy element.

8 ounces extra-firm
   tofu, drained
¼ cup lemon juice
2 tablespoons olive oil
2 tablespoons
   dried oregano
1 teaspoon freshly ground
   black pepper
2 garlic cloves, minced
8 sourdough bread slices
1 avocado, sliced
4 lettuce leaves

1. Slice the tofu into eight slabs.

2. In a small bowl, mix together the lemon juice, oil, oregano, pepper, and garlic. Add the tofu and set aside to marinate for 15 minutes, or cover and marinate in the refrigerator overnight.

3. Heat a medium skillet over medium heat. Working in batches, place the tofu in the skillet in a single layer (reserve the marinade for drizzling) and cook for 5 to 10 minutes, until golden brown on both sides.

4. While the tofu is cooking, toast the bread.

5. Assemble the sandwiches with avocado, lettuce, and tofu pieces. Drizzle the marinade over the cooked tofu for extra flavor.

Per serving (1 sandwich): Calories: 377; Protein: 14g; Total Fat: 19g; Saturated Fat: 3g; Total Carbohydrates: 41g; Fiber: 6g; Cholesterol: 0mg; Phosphorus: 181mg; Potassium: 470mg; Sodium: 395mg; Sugar: 4g

Tzatziki Egg Salad Sandwich

STAGE 5

Serves 4 / Prep time: 15 minutes / **Cook time:** 10 minutes

Egg salad is a sandwich staple that is super easy to make. This recipe features yogurt instead of saturated fat–laden mayonnaise for a healthier—but still flavorful—spin on the classic.

3 large eggs

½ cup Tzatziki Sauce (page 113), plus more for serving, if desired

½ cup diced celery

1 teaspoon freshly ground black pepper

8 sourdough bread slices

4 lettuce leaves

4 tomato slices

1. Place the eggs in a small pot and add water to cover. Bring the water to a boil over high heat, then cook the eggs for 9 minutes. With a slotted spoon, remove the eggs from the pot and place them in a bowl of ice and water to cool.

2. When cool enough to handle, peel and dice the eggs and put them in a small bowl. Add the ½ cup tzatziki sauce, celery, and pepper.

3. Assemble each sandwich with ¼ cup of the egg salad, a lettuce leaf, and a slice of tomato. Top with extra tzatziki sauce, if desired, before adding the second slice of bread.

Per serving (1 sandwich): Calories: 408; Protein: 19g; Total Fat: 7g; Saturated Fat: 2g; Total Carbohydrates: 68g; Fiber: 3g; Cholesterol: 140mg; Phosphorus: 220mg; Potassium: 306mg; Sodium: 435mg; Sugar: 7g

Lemon-Dill Chickpea Salad Sandwich

STAGE 5

Serves 4 / Prep time: 10 minutes

This quick-and-easy plant-based sandwich is satisfying—and packed with protein. The delicious flavors of lemon and dill come together to make a sandwich that is packed with flavor and portable, ideal for taking to work or to dialysis.

2 (15-ounce) cans no-added-salt chickpeas, drained and rinsed

3 tablespoons lemon juice

4 teaspoons olive oil

½ cup diced red bell pepper

2 scallions, green parts only, chopped

1 tablespoon dried dill

½ teaspoon freshly ground black pepper

4 lettuce leaves

8 sourdough bread slices

1. In a medium bowl, combine the chickpeas, lemon juice, and oil. With a potato masher or fork, mash the chickpeas until they start to come together and become creamy.

2. Add the bell pepper, scallions, dill, and pepper to the chickpea mixture and stir to combine.

3. Divide the chickpea mixture and lettuce evenly among four slices of the bread, close the sandwiches, and enjoy.

TIP: Choose canned rather than dried chickpeas. They are convenient and lower in potassium.

Per serving (1 sandwich): Calories: 393; Protein: 23g; Total Fat: 8g; Saturated Fat: 1g; Total Carbohydrates: 57g; Fiber: 10g; Cholesterol: 0mg; Phosphorus: 206mg; Potassium: 342mg; Sodium: 444mg; Sugar: 8g

Chickpea Noodle Soup

STAGE 5

Serves 10 / Prep time: 5 minutes / **Cook time:** 20 minutes

With chickpeas replacing chicken, and orzo for the noodles, this dish is a plant-based twist on a classic. It's a comforting, cure-all-for-everything bowl of soup that is ready to serve in less than 30 minutes! It may become your go-to on a fall or winter day to warm you up.

2 tablespoons olive oil

1 medium white onion, chopped

1 cup chopped celery

1 cup chopped carrots

10 cups no-added-salt vegetable broth

2 teaspoons freshly ground black pepper

2 (15-ounce) cans no-added-salt chickpeas, drained and rinsed

8 ounces orzo

Chopped fresh herbs, for garnish (optional)

1. In a large stockpot, heat the oil over medium heat. Add the onion, celery, and carrots and cook, stirring, until the onion is translucent and soft, about 5 minutes.

2. Add the broth, pepper, and chickpeas and raise the heat to high to bring the broth to a boil.

3. Reduce the heat to medium, add the orzo, and simmer for 5 minutes, or until the orzo is tender.

4. Garnish with fresh herbs, if desired, and serve warm.

TIP: To freeze the soup, let it cool, then transfer it to zip-top bags or airtight containers and freeze for up to 3 months.

Per serving (1¼ cups) Calories: 182; Protein: 8g; Total Fat: 4g; Saturated Fat: 0g; Total Carbohydrates: 30g; Fiber: 5g; Cholesterol: 0mg; Phosphorus: 140mg; Potassium: 267mg; Sodium: 114mg; Sugar: 5g

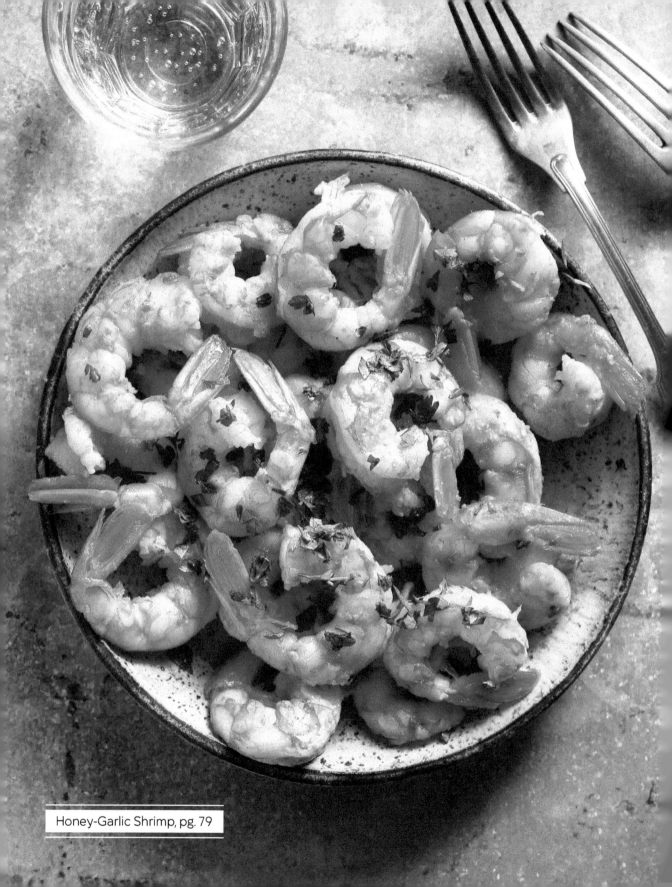

Honey-Garlic Shrimp, pg. 79

Fish and Seafood

Tuna Avocado Wrap

STAGES 1–3

Serves 4 / Prep time: 15 minutes

This wrap is versatile, fresh, and packed full of flavor from the pickled vegetables and tuna. An affordable protein, canned albacore also provides ample omega-3s and vitamin D. Remember to read food labels and choose a low-sodium canned tuna.

2 (5-ounce) cans low-sodium
   albacore tuna in
   water, drained
1 small avocado
1 tablespoon lemon juice
¼ cup chopped celery
2 tablespoons chopped
   red onion
1 teaspoon red
   pepper flakes
4 lettuce leaves
½ cup sliced yellow
   bell pepper
4 (6-inch) low-sodium corn
   tortillas
Pickled Vegetables
   (page 114)

1. In a medium bowl, mash together the tuna, avocado, and lemon juice until combined. Add the celery, onion, and red pepper flakes. Mix well to combine.

2. To assemble the wraps, top each tortilla with 1 lettuce leaf, one-quarter of the tuna mixture, and 2 tablespoons of the bell pepper. Top with pickled vegetables, tightly roll up each tortilla, and serve.

TIP: Light tuna (or skipjack tuna) is a great low-mercury alternative to albacore.

Per serving (1 wrap): Calories: 223; Protein: 16g; Total Fat: 10g; Saturated Fat: 2g; Total Carbohydrates: 19g; Fiber: 5g; Cholesterol: 24mg; Phosphorus: 245mg; Potassium: 478mg; Sodium: 227mg; Sugar: 1g

Tuna Ceviche

STAGES 1–3

Serves 4 / Prep time: 10 minutes

Ceviche is a South American dish of raw fish cured in citrus juices. This twist on ceviche uses canned tuna because it's easy to work with and more practical to prepare. If you have time, prepare the ceviche an hour in advance and let the flavors meld together.

2 (5-ounce) cans low-sodium albacore tuna in water, drained

1 small avocado, diced

½ cup chopped cherry tomatoes

2 teaspoons dried dill

⅛ teaspoon ground cumin

1 teaspoon red pepper flakes

2 tablespoons lime juice

½ teaspoon olive oil

4 cups arugula

1. In a medium bowl, mix together the tuna, avocado, tomatoes, dill, cumin, red pepper flakes, lime juice, and oil.

2. Divide the arugula evenly among four plates and top each with an equal amount of the tuna ceviche.

TIP: This dish goes nicely with flavors that complement the citrus, such as corn, sweet potatoes, or plantains. Remember to choose low-potassium accompaniments, if needed.

Per serving (½ cup): Calories: 149; Protein: 13g; Total Fat: 9g; Saturated Fat: 1g; Total Carbohydrates: 7g; Fiber: 4g; Cholesterol: 20mg; Phosphorus: 125mg; Potassium: 467mg; Sodium: 151mg; Sugar: 1g

Sweet-and-Spicy Shrimp

STAGES 1–3

Serves 4 / Prep time: 20 minutes / **Cook time:** 15 minutes

Sweet chili sauce, sometimes referred to as Thai or Asian sweet chili sauce, is a combination of sweet, savory, tangy, and spicy flavors. This marinated shrimp dish finds the perfect balance of sweet and heat to excite your taste buds and fill your belly. For this recipe you will need four wooden or metal skewers.

¼ cup Sweet Chili Sauce (page 117)

1 pound raw shrimp (medium size), peeled and deveined

1 tablespoon olive oil

½ cup sliced white onion

2 yellow bell peppers, sliced

1 cup broccoli florets

1. If using wooden skewers, soak them in water for 30 minutes before using to prevent burning.

2. Marinate the shrimp in the sweet chili sauce for 10 minutes.

3. Thread 4 to 6 shrimp through the tail onto each skewer.

4. Heat a medium skillet over medium heat. Add the skewers and cook for 3 to 4 minutes per side, until the shrimp are pink in color and opaque. Remove from the heat.

5. In a second medium skillet, heat the oil over medium heat. Add the onion, bell peppers, and broccoli and cook, stirring, until tender, 5 to 8 minutes.

6. Serve the vegetables with the shrimp.

Per serving (1 skewer and 1 cup vegetables): Calories: 159; Protein: 24g; Total Fat: 4g; Saturated Fat: 1g; Total Carbohydrates: 7g; Fiber: 1g; Cholesterol: 183mg; Phosphorus: 276mg; Potassium: 487mg; Sodium: 141mg; Sugar: 1g

Cod Tacos

STAGES 1–3

Serves 4 / Prep time: 5 minutes / **Cook time:** 10 minutes

Cod is a great protein, and because it is lower in potassium and phosphorus than other white fish, it is kidney-friendly. This speedy supper is made in less than 20 minutes in just one pan, making it perfect for a busy weeknight.

8 ounces skinless cod, cut into cubes

2 teaspoons Mexican Seasoning (page 120)

1 tablespoon olive oil, divided

3 bell peppers (red, orange, and yellow), sliced

1 yellow onion, sliced

8 (6-inch) low-sodium corn tortillas

1. In a medium bowl, toss the cod in the Mexican seasoning to coat well.

2. In a medium skillet, heat ½ tablespoon of the oil over medium heat. Add the bell peppers and onion and cook for 5 to 8 minutes, until the vegetables are tender. Transfer the vegetables to a bowl and set aside.

3. Add the remaining ½ tablespoon oil and the cod to the skillet and cook over medium heat for 2 to 3 minutes, until the underside is golden. Flip the cod and cook for 2 to 3 minutes more, until the fish is tender and flakes easily with a fork.

4. Serve the cod and vegetables in the tortillas.

TIP: Try adding some Pickled Vegetables (page 114) for a tangy twist.

Per serving (2 tacos): Calories: 223; Protein: 13g; Total Fat: 5g; Saturated Fat: 1g; Total Carbohydrates: 32g; Fiber: 5g; Cholesterol: 27mg; Phosphorus: 354mg; Potassium: 442mg; Sodium: 182mg; Sugar: 5g

Lemon-Garlic Cod

STAGES 1–3

Serves 4 / Prep time: 10 minutes **/ Cook time:** 20 minutes

Cod is a mild-tasting fish that pairs well with any flavors with which it is cooked. This lemon-garlic cod is served with parboiled rice, a low-glycemic-index carbohydrate that does not spike blood glucose levels as quickly as other types of white rice.

1 cup parboiled rice

Nonstick cooking spray

4 (2-ounce) skinless
 cod fillets

2 teaspoons unsalted butter

1 tablespoon olive oil

3 garlic cloves, minced

3 tablespoons lemon juice

2 teaspoons dried oregano

2 cups green beans, cut into
 1-inch lengths

1. Prepare the rice as directed on the package. Set aside.

2. Preheat the oven to 400°F. Coat a baking dish with nonstick spray. Bring a large pot of water to a boil.

3. Place the cod in the prepared baking dish.

4. In a small nonstick saucepan, combine the butter, oil, garlic, lemon juice, and oregano and heat over medium heat for 2 minutes. Remove from the heat.

5. Drizzle the butter mixture over the cod. Bake for 12 to 15 minutes, until the fish is tender and flakes easily with a fork.

6. While the fish is cooking, blanch the green beans in the boiling water for 2 minutes. Drain, then place in a bowl of ice and water for 1 minute to stop the cooking; drain again before serving.

7. Serve the fish with the rice and green beans.

TIP: This dish is also great with other low-potassium kidney-friendly whole grain options such as couscous, bulgur, or barley.

Per serving (1 cod fillet, ¾ cup rice, and ½ cup green beans): Calories: 279; Protein: 21g; Total Fat: 6g; Saturated Fat: 2g; Total Carbohydrates: 34g; Fiber: 3g; Cholesterol: 60mg; Phosphorus: 375mg; Potassium: 433mg; Sodium: 358mg; Sugar: 2g

Orange-Ginger Salmon

STAGES 1–3

Serves 4 / Prep time: 5 minutes / **Cook time:** 20 minutes

This sweet-and-tangy salmon dish will get your taste buds excited for more. This recipe is quick to pull together for a weeknight meal and is packed with lots of heart-healthy omega-3 fats from the salmon.

¼ cup honey

¼ cup orange juice

2 tablespoons minced fresh ginger

2 garlic cloves, minced

1 tablespoon low-sodium soy sauce

4 (2-ounce) skinless salmon fillets

1. Preheat the oven to 400°F. Line a baking sheet with parchment paper.

2. In a small bowl, stir together the honey, orange juice, ginger, garlic, and soy sauce.

3. Place the salmon on the prepared baking sheet and drizzle with the honey mixture.

4. Bake for 12 to 15 minutes, until the salmon is tender and flakes easily with a fork, then switch the oven to broil and broil the fish for 3 minutes.

TIP: This recipe can be sticky because of the honey. Lining your baking sheet with parchment paper makes cleanup easy.

Per serving (1 salmon fillet): Calories: 159; Protein: 12g; Total Fat: 4g; Saturated Fat: 0g; Total Carbohydrates: 20g; Fiber: 0g; Cholesterol: 31mg; Phosphorus: 126mg; Potassium: 348mg; Sodium: 154mg; Sugar: 19g

Chile-Lime Salmon Bowls

STAGES 1–3

Serves 4 / Prep time: 10 minutes / **Cook time:** 35 minutes

These salmon bowls are great year-round. The salmon soaks up the spices in this recipe, meaning these bowls are packed with flavor! Lime is a great addition for a pop of citrus and vitamin C, which can help boost the immune system.

1 cup parboiled rice

4 (2-ounce) skinless
   salmon fillets

1 tablespoon low-sodium
   soy sauce

2 tablespoons olive
   oil, divided

1 teaspoon paprika

2 teaspoons garlic powder

2 teaspoons onion powder

1 cup broccoli florets

2 cups cauliflower florets

1 cup sliced orange
   bell pepper

Spicy Sauce (page 115)

1 lime, cut into wedges,
   for serving

1. Cook the rice as directed on the package. Set aside to cool.

2. Preheat the oven to 400°F. Line a baking sheet with parchment paper.

3. Place the salmon on the prepared baking sheet.

4. In a small bowl, whisk together the soy sauce, 1 tablespoon of the oil, the paprika, garlic powder, and onion powder. Drizzle the sauce over the salmon. Bake for 12 to 15 minutes, until the fish is tender and flakes easily with a fork, then switch the oven to broil and broil the fish for 3 minutes.

5. While the salmon bakes, in a medium skillet, heat the remaining 1 tablespoon oil over medium heat. Add the broccoli, cauliflower, and bell pepper and cook, stirring, until the vegetables are tender, 6 to 8 minutes.

6. Divide the rice evenly among four bowls. Top each with a salmon fillet and 1 cup of the vegetables. Drizzle with the spicy sauce and serve with the lime wedges alongside for squeezing over the top.

Per serving (1 salmon fillet, ¾ cup rice, 1 cup vegetables):
Calories: 315; Protein: 16g; Total Fat: 11g; Saturated Fat: 2g;
Total Carbohydrates: 38g; Fiber: 3g; Cholesterol: 31mg;
Phosphorus: 206mg; Potassium: 575mg; Sodium: 181mg; Sugar: 2g

Salmon Salad with Tzatziki

STAGES 1–3

Serves 4 / Prep time: 15 minutes

A perfect dish for summer, this chopped salad is packed with nutrients and will fill you up. Creamy, tangy tzatziki, a traditional Greek dip, serves as the dressing.

1 (7.5-ounce) can boneless salmon, drained

1 tablespoon olive oil

1 teaspoon dried dill

½ teaspoon freshly ground black pepper

1 head lettuce, coarsely chopped

1 cup cherry tomatoes, halved

1 medium yellow bell pepper, sliced

Tzatziki Sauce (page 113)

1. In a small bowl, mix the salmon, oil, dill, and pepper.

2. Divide the lettuce evenly among four bowls. Top each evenly with the tomatoes, bell pepper, and salmon mixture. Drizzle the tzatziki on top and enjoy.

Per serving (¼ cup salmon and ¼ salad): Calories: 115; Protein: 11g; Total Fat: 6g; Saturated Fat: 1g; Total Carbohydrates: 6g; Fiber: 4g; Cholesterol: 35mg; Phosphorus: 196mg; Potassium: 381mg; Sodium: 167mg; Sugar: 2g

Garlic-Butter Crab Pasta

STAGES 1–3

Serves 4 / Prep time: 5 minutes / **Cook time:** 20 minutes

This pasta is one of the quickest and tastiest dishes you'll ever prepare. It is restaurant-quality and so delicious you'll want to eat it out of the pan.

4 ounces orzo

1 tablespoon olive oil

1 small white onion, diced

4 garlic cloves, minced

1 medium red bell
  pepper, diced

2 tablespoons
  dried oregano

1 teaspoon freshly ground
  black pepper

1 tablespoon
  unsalted butter

1 tablespoon lemon juice

4 (4¼-ounce) cans crabmeat

1. Cook the orzo as directed on the package. Set aside.

2. In a medium skillet, heat the oil over medium heat. Add the onion, garlic, and bell pepper and cook until the vegetables are tender and the onion is translucent, about 3 minutes.

3. Add the oregano, black pepper, butter, lemon juice, and crabmeat and stir to combine.

4. Add the cooked orzo and stir until all the ingredients are incorporated, then cook until warmed through, about 3 minutes.

5. Remove the skillet from the heat and serve.

Per serving (2 cups): Calories: 303; Protein: 19g; Total Fat: 7g; Saturated Fat: 3g; Total Carbohydrates: 34g; Fiber: 3g; Cholesterol: 104mg; Phosphorus: 302mg; Potassium: 413mg; Sodium: 482mg; Sugar: 1g

Spicy Tuna Bowls

STAGE 4

Serves 4 / Prep time: 20 minutes **/ Cook time:** 20 minutes

These bowls are an homage to a spicy tuna hand roll, but use cooked canned fish. Individuals with CKD should avoid sushi made with raw fish, as raw fish may contain parasites that can cause infection.

1 cup parboiled rice

2 (5-ounce) cans low-sodium
   skipjack tuna in
   water, drained

1 cup sliced cucumber

1 cup shredded carrots

1 small avocado, diced

Spicy Sauce (page 115)

Pickled Vegetables
   (page 114)

1. Cook the rice as directed on the package. Set aside to cool.

2. Divide the cooled rice evenly among four bowls. Top each evenly with one-quarter of the tuna, cucumber, carrots, and avocado. Drizzle with the spicy sauce and serve with pickled vegetables.

Per serving (½ cup rice, ⅓ cup tuna, ¼ cup cucumber, ¼ cup carrot, and ¼ avocado): Calories: 296; Protein: 17g; Total Fat: 9g; Saturated Fat: 2g; Total Carbohydrates: 36g; Fiber: 5g; Cholesterol: 24mg; Phosphorus: 190mg; Potassium: 492mg; Sodium: 239mg; Sugar: 2g

Lemon-Pepper Salmon

STAGE 4

Serves 4 / Prep time: 5 minutes **/ Cook time:** 20 minutes

This is a foolproof recipe if you or your loved one is in the mood for something that will knock your taste buds off and fill your belly. The salmon tastes great with roasted cauliflower and green beans, which can be cooked on the same pan for an effortless, balanced meal.

1 lemon, thinly sliced

4 (2-ounce) skinless salmon fillets

¼ cup lemon juice

2 teaspoons dried dill

2 teaspoons freshly ground black pepper

1 tablespoon olive oil

1. Preheat the oven to 400°F. Line a baking sheet with parchment paper.

2. Place half the lemons on the prepared baking sheet and place the salmon fillets on top.

3. In a small bowl, stir together the lemon juice, dill, pepper, and oil. Drizzle over the salmon and top with the remaining lemon slices.

4. Bake for 12 to 15 minutes, until the salmon is tender and flakes easily with a fork, then switch the oven to broil and broil the fish for 3 minutes.

Per serving (1 salmon fillet): Calories: 122; Protein: 12g; Total Fat: 7g; Saturated Fat: 1g; Total Carbohydrates: 2g; Fiber: 0g; Cholesterol: 26mg; Phosphorus: 154mg; Potassium: 280mg; Sodium: 27mg; Sugar: 1g

Honey-Garlic Shrimp

STAGE 5

Serves 4 / Prep time: 10 minutes / **Cook time:** 10 minutes

This recipe looks and tastes like the kind of meal you'd get at a high-quality restaurant, but comes together quickly at home with just a few ingredients. Serve it with your favorite stir-fried vegetables, rice, or couscous, or over a salad.

¼ cup honey

2 tablespoons low-sodium soy sauce

2 teaspoons minced garlic

1 teaspoon minced fresh ginger

1 teaspoon olive oil

1 pound raw shrimp, peeled and deveined

1 lemon, cut into wedges, for serving

1. In a small bowl, stir together the honey, soy sauce, garlic, and ginger.

2. Put the shrimp in a medium bowl and pour over half the marinade (reserve the remaining marinade for serving). Set aside to marinate for 10 minutes.

3. In a medium skillet, heat the oil over medium heat. Add the shrimp and cook for 2 to 3 minutes per side, until pink in color and opaque.

4. Remove the shrimp from the skillet and toss in the reserved marinade. Serve hot, with the lemon wedges for squeezing on top.

Per serving (¼ of the shrimp): Calories: 179; Protein: 24g; Total Fat: 2g; Saturated Fat: 0g; Total Carbohydrates: 19g; Fiber: 0g; Cholesterol: 183mg; Phosphorus: 259mg; Potassium: 355mg; Sodium: 392mg; Sugar: 18g

Sheet Pan Cod with Roasted Bell Pepper and Broccolini

STAGE 5

Serves 4 / Prep time: 5 minutes / **Cook time:** 20 minutes

Sheet pan meals are ideal for weeknights because they make both cooking and cleanup quick and simple. The vegetables in this recipe help the body maintain its acid-base balance, are great sources of antioxidants and fiber, and give this dish a pop of color.

2½ tablespoons Greek Seasoning (page 120)

3 tablespoons olive oil

3 tablespoons lemon juice

1 bunch broccolini, bottom ½ inch trimmed

2 orange bell peppers, sliced

2 cups green beans

4 (3-ounce) skinless cod fillets

1. Preheat the oven to 425°F. Line a baking sheet with parchment paper.

2. In a medium bowl, whisk together the Greek seasoning, oil, and lemon juice.

3. Add the broccolini, bell peppers, and green beans to the bowl and toss to combine. Place the vegetables over one half of the prepared baking sheet, reserving any marinade left in the bowl. Place the cod on the other half of the baking sheet and drizzle with the remaining marinade.

4. Roast for 20 minutes, until the fish is tender and flakes easily with a fork.

Per serving (1 fillet and 2 cups vegetables): Calories: 199; Protein: 15g; Total Fat: 11g; Saturated Fat: 2g; Total Carbohydrates: 10g; Fiber: 2g; Cholesterol: 40mg; Phosphorus: 276mg; Potassium: 493mg; Sodium: 262mg; Sugar: 2g

Crab Cakes

STAGE 5

Serves 4 / Prep time: 10 minutes / **Cook time:** 10 minutes

Crab cakes, with their sweet, juicy meat and dab of sauce, are a delicacy. This recipe uses oats to bind the ingredients and help the crab cakes hold their shape. The oats also give the crab cakes a golden crust and add a bit of fiber to the meal.

4 (4¼-ounce) cans crab-
  meat, drained
2 scallions, green parts
  only, chopped
2 tablespoons low-fat plain
  Greek yogurt
1½ cups rolled
  (old-fashioned) oats
1 tablespoon lemon juice
1 large egg, beaten
2 teaspoons dried dill
1 teaspoon freshly ground
  black pepper
1 tablespoon olive oil
Tzatziki Sauce (page 113)

1. In a medium bowl, gently stir together the crab-meat, scallions, yogurt, oats, lemon juice, egg, dill, and pepper to combine. Form the mixture into four patties.

2. In a medium skillet, heat the oil over medium heat. Add the crab cakes and cook for 2 to 3 minutes, until golden brown on the bottom, then flip and cook for 2 to 3 minutes more, until golden brown on the second side.

3. Serve with the tzatziki for dipping.

TIP: This dish tastes great with a side of salad or coleslaw.

Per serving (1 crab cake): Calories: 293; Protein: 27g; Total Fat: 8g; Saturated Fat: 2g; Total Carbohydrates: 25g; Fiber: 4g; Cholesterol: 151mg; Phosphorus: 469mg; Potassium: 481mg; Sodium: 498mg; Sugar: 1g

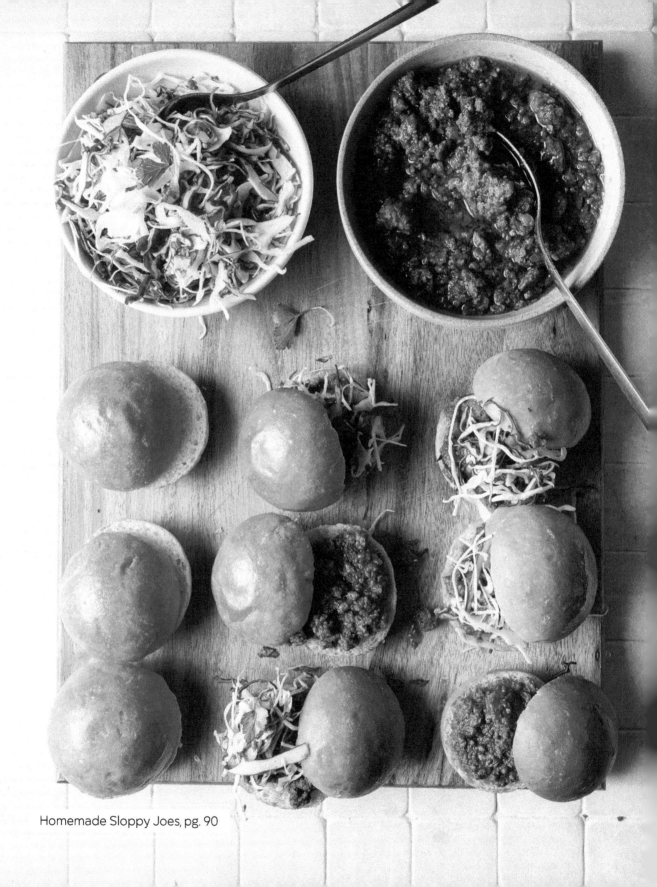

Homemade Sloppy Joes, pg. 90

CHAPTER SIX

Poultry and Meat

Citrus and Herb Turkey Breast

STAGES 1–3

Serves 4 / Prep time: 15 minutes **/ Cook time:** 10 minutes

Turkey can be dry and bland, but this recipe always comes out moist and flavorful. Turkey has many great nutrients, like niacin, selenium, vitamin B_6, and zinc, so it is a great addition to a kidney-friendly diet. Serve this turkey with couscous and roasted carrots and parsnips alongside.

2½ tablespoons Greek Seasoning (page 120)

¼ cup lemon juice

8 ounces boneless, skinless turkey breast, cut into 4 (2-ounce) cutlets

1 tablespoon olive oil

1. In a medium bowl, combine the Greek seasoning and lemon juice. Add the turkey and set aside to marinate for 10 minutes.

2. In a medium skillet, heat the oil over medium-high heat. Add the turkey cutlets and cook until golden brown on the bottom, 2 to 3 minutes, then flip and cook for 2 to 4 minutes more, until no longer pink inside. Remove from the heat and serve.

TIP: Looking for a low-sodium way to flavor your holiday turkey? This marinade is a great option: Slather it all over your bird and let it sit for 15 minutes before roasting.

Per serving (1 cutlet): Calories: 97; Protein: 13g; Total Fat: 4g; Saturated Fat: 1g; Total Carbohydrates: 1g; Fiber: 0g; Cholesterol: 38mg; Phosphorus: 109mg; Potassium: 149mg; Sodium: 67mg; Sugar: 0g

Turkey Kofta with Tahini

STAGES 1–3

Serves 4 / Prep time: 10 minutes **/ Cook time:** 15 minutes

Kofta (or kefta) are Middle Eastern spiced meatballs typically made with lamb or beef. This recipe uses turkey, a leaner protein choice, but it's still packed with flavor. The kofta are served with a delicious homemade tahini sauce, which imparts the rich, nutty flavor of sesame.

10 ounces 93% lean
   ground turkey

¼ cup minced white onion

2 garlic cloves, minced

¼ cup rolled
   (old-fashioned) oats

½ teaspoon ground cumin

½ teaspoon paprika

4 lettuce leaves, chopped

8 cherry tomatoes, halved

½ cup sliced cucumber

¼ cup sliced white onion

Tahini Sauce (page 112)

2 (8-inch) pita pockets,
   halved

1. Preheat the oven to 450°F. Line a baking sheet with parchment paper.

2. In a medium bowl, combine the turkey, minced onion, garlic, oats, cumin, and paprika and gently knead with your hands to combine. Divide the mixture into eight portions and form each into an oblong oval.

3. Place the kofta on the prepared baking sheet and bake for 12 to 15 minutes, until the juices run clear and the inside is no longer pink.

4. Divide the lettuce, tomato, cucumber, and sliced onion evenly among four plates. Top each with 2 kofta, drizzle with the tahini sauce, and serve with the pitas on the side.

Per serving (2 kofta, ½ pita, and 1 cup vegetables): Calories: 229; Protein: 18g; Total Fat: 7g; Saturated Fat: 2g; Total Carbohydrates: 24g; Fiber: 2g; Cholesterol: 52mg; Phosphorus: 217mg; Potassium: 387mg; Sodium: 214mg; Sugar: 2g

Cilantro-Lime Chicken

STAGES 1–3

Serves 4 / Prep time: 20 minutes **/ Cook time:** 10 minutes

Cilantro has a complex citrusy flavor, but depending on your genetics, you may find it to be too pungent. If you're not a fan of cilantro, use parsley or basil in this dish instead. This chicken is best enjoyed alongside roasted potatoes or rice and green beans.

1 bunch cilantro

½ cup lime juice

4 garlic cloves

2 tablespoons olive oil, divided

1½ teaspoons ground cumin

1 teaspoon red pepper flakes

½ teaspoon freshly ground black pepper

8 ounces boneless, skinless chicken thighs

1. In a food processor or blender, combine the cilantro, lime juice, garlic, 1 tablespoon of the oil, the cumin, red pepper flakes, and black pepper and puree until smooth. Transfer to a medium bowl and add the chicken thighs. Stir until well coated. Cover the bowl with plastic wrap and marinate the chicken in the refrigerator for at least 15 minutes or up to 48 hours.

2. In a medium skillet, heat the remaining 1 tablespoon oil over medium heat. Add the chicken and cook for 8 to 10 minutes, flipping once halfway through, until the chicken is no longer pink inside and the juices run clear.

TIP: The best part about this dish is that the longer you marinate the chicken, the more flavor you'll get.

Per serving (2 ounces): Calories: 143; Protein: 11g; Total Fat: 9g; Saturated Fat: 2g; Total Carbohydrates: 4g; Fiber: 0g; Cholesterol: 52mg; Phosphorus: 117mg; Potassium: 217mg; Sodium: 59mg; Sugar: 1g

Pineapple Chicken Thighs

STAGES 1–3

*Serves 4 / **Prep time:** 5 minutes / **Cook time:** 25 minutes*

This recipe changes things up by using chicken thighs instead of breasts, which adds richness and moisture to the dish for a treat of sweet and savory flavors. Enjoy this stir-fry dish served over rice.

1 cup parboiled rice

1 tablespoon olive oil

1 red bell pepper, sliced

1 medium white onion, sliced

5 ounces boneless, skinless chicken thighs, cut into cubes

1 teaspoon cornstarch

½ teaspoon water

1 (8-ounce) can unsweetened pineapple chunks in 100% juice

2 tablespoons low-sodium soy sauce

1. Cook the rice as directed on the package. Set aside.

2. In a medium skillet, heat the oil over medium heat. Add the bell pepper and onion and cook, stirring, until the vegetables are tender, about 5 minutes. Remove the vegetables from the skillet and set aside.

3. Add the chicken to the skillet and cook over medium heat until cooked through and no longer pink inside, about 10 minutes. Remove the chicken from the skillet and set it aside with the vegetables.

4. In a small bowl, mix the cornstarch and water to create a slurry. In the same skillet, combine the pineapple, soy sauce, and cornstarch slurry and stir to combine. Let the mixture bubble over medium heat until slightly thickened, 5 to 7 minutes.

5. Return the vegetables and chicken to the skillet and stir to coat with the pineapple sauce. Cook briefly, until the chicken is well coated and the sauce is warmed through.

6. Serve the chicken and vegetables over the rice.

Per serving (¾ cup rice, 1¼ ounces chicken, and ½ cup vegetables): Calories: 262; Protein: 11g; Total Fat: 5g; Saturated Fat: 1g; Total Carbohydrates: 43g; Fiber: 3g; Cholesterol: 32mg; Phosphorus: 119mg; Potassium: 308mg; Sodium: 295mg; Sugar: 11g

Honey-Garlic BBQ Chicken

STAGES 1–3

Serves 4 / Prep time: 10 minutes **/ Cook time:** 20 minutes

This recipe uses pantry staples to transform chicken into a meal to remember. Using homemade BBQ sauce results in moist, flavorful chicken every time. Serve this dish with couscous and a salad alongside.

2 tablespoons olive oil, divided

6 ounces boneless, skinless chicken thighs

4 garlic cloves, minced

¼ cup BBQ Sauce (page 116)

¼ cup honey

1 teaspoon red pepper flakes

1. In a medium skillet, heat 1 tablespoon of the oil over medium heat. Add the chicken and cook for 8 to 10 minutes, flipping once halfway through, until the juices run clear and the chicken is no longer pink inside. Remove the chicken from the skillet and set aside.

2. In a small saucepan, combine the remaining 1 tablespoon oil and the garlic. Cook over medium heat until the garlic softens, 1 to 2 minutes. Add the BBQ sauce, honey, and red pepper flakes and simmer for 5 minutes.

3. Transfer the sauce to a medium bowl, add the chicken, and mix until well coated.

Per serving (½ cup): Calories: 210; Protein: 9g; Total Fat: 9g; Saturated Fat: 1g; Total Carbohydrates: 26g; Fiber: 0g; Cholesterol: 39mg; Phosphorus: 86mg; Potassium: 166mg; Sodium: 226mg; Sugar: 23g

Red Wine Vinegar Baked Chicken Breast

STAGES 1–3

Serves 4 / Prep time: 5 minutes / **Cook time:** 20 minutes

Inspired by a classic French dish called *poulet au vinaigre* (chicken with vinegar), this recipe gets its tangy flavor from red wine vinegar. Shallots, a cousin of onion with a softer and more delicate flavor, are a great addition. You can substitute shallots in any recipe that calls for onions.

8 ounces boneless, skinless chicken breasts, chopped

1 teaspoon freshly ground black pepper

½ cup red wine vinegar

1½ teaspoons honey

½ cup no-added-salt vegetable broth

1½ teaspoons tomato paste

1 tablespoon olive oil

2 shallots, finely chopped

2 garlic cloves, minced

1 tablespoon low-fat plain Greek yogurt

1. Season the chicken on both sides with pepper.

2. In a medium saucepan, combine the vinegar, honey, broth, and tomato paste and mix to combine. Bring the mixture to a boil over medium-high heat, then reduce the heat to maintain a simmer and cook for 5 minutes, or until it reduces by about half. Remove the saucepan from the heat.

3. In a large skillet, heat the olive oil over medium heat. Add the chicken and cook for about 10 minutes, until it's cooked through and no longer pink inside. Remove the chicken from the skillet and set aside.

4. In the same skillet, combine the shallots and garlic and cook over medium heat until soft, about 3 minutes. Add the sauce, bring to a boil, and simmer for 5 minutes. Remove from the heat.

5. Return the chicken to the pan. Add the yogurt and stir to combine, then serve.

TIP: This dish is best served with green beans, parboiled rice, or couscous, which is a low-potassium carbohydrate option.

Per serving (2 ounces): Calories: 115; Protein: 13g; Total Fat: 4g; Saturated Fat: 1g; Total Carbohydrates: 4g; Fiber: 0g; Cholesterol: 33mg; Phosphorus: 140mg; Potassium: 205mg; Sodium: 181mg; Sugar: 3g

Homemade Sloppy Joes

STAGES 1–3

Serves 6 / Prep time: 5 minutes / **Cook time:** 20 minutes

Who else was raised on sloppy Joes? Sloppy Joes are a childhood memory and comfort food for many. This adult version is kidney-friendly and packs a bit more flavor with a homemade low- sodium sauce. To add some crunch, serve the sandwiches with shredded red cabbage.

8 ounces 93% lean
   ground beef

1 tablespoon olive oil

1 red bell pepper, diced

1 medium white onion, diced

1 cup shredded carrots

12 ounces low-sodium
   tomato sauce

2 tablespoons sugar

2 teaspoons garlic powder

2 teaspoons paprika

1 teaspoon freshly ground
   black pepper

6 brioche buns or
   12 slider rolls

1. In a medium stockpot, brown the beef, breaking it up with a wooden spoon as it cooks, until it's cooked thoroughly and no longer pink, 5 to 8 minutes. Drain the grease from the beef, then return the meat to the pot.

2. Add the oil, bell pepper, onion, and carrots and cook until the vegetables are tender, about 5 minutes.

3. Add the tomato sauce, sugar, garlic powder, paprika, and black pepper to the pot and stir until everything is well combined. Bring the mixture to a simmer, then cook for 5 minutes. Remove from the heat.

4. Serve on the buns.

TIP: You can easily substitute no-added-salt canned lentils (drained and rinsed) for the ground beef to create a plant-based sloppy Joe.

Per serving (½ cup meat mixture and 1 bun): Calories: 242; Protein: 14g; Total Fat: 6g; Saturated Fat: 2g; Total Carbohydrates: 34g; Fiber: 3g; Cholesterol: 23mg; Phosphorus: 159mg; Potassium: 490mg; Sodium: 257mg; Sugar: 11g

Ginger Beef

STAGES 1–3

Serves 4 / Prep time: 10 minutes / **Cook time:** 20 minutes

There's no need to order out when you can make amazing ginger beef at home! This recipe is great for weeknights, and the skirt or flank steak can be swapped out for cheaper cuts of beef, such as top round or beef shoulder.

1 cup parboiled rice

1 tablespoon olive oil

1 medium white onion, sliced

1 cup sliced orange bell pepper

1 cup broccoli florets

4 garlic cloves, minced

2 tablespoons finely chopped fresh ginger

8 ounces skirt steak or flank steak, thinly sliced across the grain

2 tablespoons low-sodium soy sauce

½ teaspoon red pepper flakes

1 tablespoon honey

1 tablespoon red wine vinegar

1. Cook the rice as directed on the package. Set aside.

2. In a medium skillet, heat the oil over medium heat. Add the onion, bell peppers, and broccoli and cook, stirring, until tender, about 5 minutes. Add the garlic and ginger and cook for 1 minute more. Remove the vegetable mixture from the skillet and set aside.

3. In the same skillet, cook the beef over medium heat for 2 to 4 minutes (it cooks quickly because the pan is preheated). Return the vegetables to skillet.

4. In a small bowl, whisk together the soy sauce, red pepper flakes, honey, and vinegar. Add the sauce to skillet and bring everything to a simmer, then cook for about 2 minutes to let the sauce thicken.

5. Serve over the rice.

TIP: Because skirt steak or flank steak are tougher cuts of meat, you need to slice them across the grain to ensure that they are tender.

Per serving (1½ cups): Calories: 299; Protein: 17g; Total Fat: 7g; Saturated Fat: 2g; Total Carbohydrates: 42g; Fiber: 3g; Cholesterol: 35mg; Phosphorus: 188mg; Potassium: 476mg; Sodium: 300mg; Sugar: 6g

Chicken Meatballs with Tahini

STAGES 1–4

Makes 12 meatballs / Prep time: 10 minutes / **Cook time:** 20 minutes

Chicken is the jack-of-all-trades in the kitchen. It can be substituted for beef or pork and is an affordable lean protein that tastes lighter compared to alternatives. These Mediterranean-inspired meatballs call for ground chicken to let the other flavors shine.

6 ounces ground chicken

1 large egg

2 garlic cloves, minced

½ cup shredded carrot

1 teaspoon ground cumin

¼ cup rolled
   (old-fashioned) oats

1 tablespoon olive oil

Tahini Sauce (page 112)

1. Preheat the oven to 375°F. Line a baking sheet with parchment paper.

2. In a large bowl, combine the chicken, egg, garlic, carrot, cumin, and oats and mix well. Shape the mixture into 1-inch balls and place them on the prepared baking sheet, evenly spaced.

3. Bake for 15 to 18 minutes, until no longer pink in the center.

4. Serve the meatballs with the tahini sauce for dipping.

TIP: Chicken is lower in saturated fat than beef and pork, making it a great heart-healthy protein.

Per serving (3 meatballs): Calories: 126; Protein: 10g; Total Fat: 8g; Saturated Fat: 2g; Total Carbohydrates: 4g; Fiber: 1g; Cholesterol: 83mg; Phosphorus: 132mg; Potassium: 315mg; Sodium: 54mg; Sugar: 1g

Sweet Chili Chicken

STAGE 4

Serves 4 / Prep time: 10 minutes / **Cook time:** 15 minutes

This recipe will have you resisting the urge to lick your plate. The secret is the sauce, which combines with moist chicken thighs for a sweet-and-spicy dish that won't disappoint. It's also a breeze to clean up, making it the perfect meal for a busy weeknight.

1 tablespoon olive oil

2 garlic cloves, minced

1 cup broccoli florets

1 red bell pepper, sliced

1 small white onion, sliced

5 ounces boneless, skinless chicken thighs, cut into cubes

¼ cup Sweet Chili Sauce (page 117)

2 tablespoons low-sodium soy sauce

1. In a medium skillet, heat the oil over medium heat. Add the garlic, broccoli, bell pepper, and onion and cook, stirring, until the vegetables are soft, about 5 minutes. Remove the vegetables from the skillet and set aside.

2. In the same skillet, cook the chicken until cooked through and no longer pink inside, about 10 minutes.

3. Add the sweet chili sauce and soy sauce and stir to coat the chicken well. Return the vegetables to the skillet and toss to combine.

TIP: This dish is best enjoyed with noodles to soak up the sauce. Try it with rice noodles or udon noodles.

Per serving (¾ cup): Calories: 120; Protein: 9g; Total Fat: 5g; Saturated Fat: 1g; Total Carbohydrates: 9g; Fiber: 3g; Cholesterol: 32mg; Phosphorus: 115mg; Potassium: 339mg; Sodium: 487mg; Sugar: 4g

Meatloaf Muffins with BBQ Sauce

STAGE 4

Serves 6 / Prep time: 10 minutes / **Cook time:** 20 minutes

This recipe is a time-saver and uses a muffin tin for individually portioned meat-loaves. Though it calls for onion, celery, and green bell pepper, you could easily use carrots, zucchini, or mushrooms instead—it's a great way to use up any excess vegetables you have in the refrigerator.

Nonstick cooking spray

8 ounces 93% lean
  ground beef

1 cup minced white onion

2 celery stalks, chopped

1 medium green bell
  pepper, chopped

1 large egg, beaten

½ cup rolled
  (old-fashioned) oats

½ cup BBQ Sauce
  (page 116), divided

3 cups green beans

1. Preheat the oven to 450°F. Coat six wells of a muffin tin with nonstick spray.

2. In a large bowl, mix the beef, onion, celery, bell pepper, egg, oats, and ¼ cup of the BBQ sauce until well combined.

3. Scoop the meat mixture evenly into the prepared wells of the muffin tin and top with the remaining ¼ cup BBQ sauce, dividing it evenly.

4. Bake the meatloaf muffins for 20 minutes, or until cooked through and no longer pink inside.

5. Meanwhile, bring a pot of water to a boil. Toward the end of the meatloaf cooking time, blanch the green beans in the boiling water for 2 minutes, then drain them and transfer to a bowl of ice and water for 1 minute to stop the cooking. Drain again and pat dry before serving alongside the meatloaf muffins.

TIP: Individually shaped uncooked meatloaf muffins, without the BBQ sauce topping, can be placed in an airtight container lined with parchment paper and frozen for up to 6 months. When ready to enjoy, thaw them in the refrigerator overnight, then top with the BBQ sauce and bake as directed. Prepare the green beans fresh just before serving.

Per serving (1 meatloaf muffin and ½ cup green beans): Calories: 125; Protein: 11g; Total Fat: 3g; Saturated Fat: 1g; Total Carbohydrates: 15g; Fiber: 3g; Cholesterol: 54mg; Phosphorus: 160mg; Potassium: 390mg; Sodium: 169mg; Sugar: 7g

Turkey Cobb Salad

STAGE 5

Serves 4 / Prep time: 10 minutes **/ Cook time:** 20 minutes

The Cobb salad is a main-dish garden salad that traditionally includes a hard-boiled egg, bacon, and chicken with a vinaigrette. This kidney-friendly alternative is packed with flavor without the salt and phosphorus of the original and features pan-seared turkey breast. It comes together to make a refreshing salad that will keep you feeling satisfied.

4 large eggs

2 tablespoons olive oil, divided

8 ounces boneless, skinless turkey breast, cut into 4 (2-ounce) cutlets

1 teaspoon freshly ground black pepper

2 tablespoons red wine vinegar

8 lettuce leaves, chopped

½ cup cherry tomatoes, halved

1 medium orange bell pepper, chopped

1. Place the eggs in a small pot and add water to cover. Bring the water to a boil over high heat, then cook the eggs for 9 minutes. With a slotted spoon, remove the eggs from the pot and transfer them to a bowl of ice and water to cool.

2. In a medium skillet, heat 1 tablespoon of the oil over medium-high heat. Season the turkey cutlets with the pepper on both sides, then add them to the pan and cook until golden brown on the bottom, 2 to 3 minutes. Flip the cutlets and cook for 2 to 4 minutes more, until they are no longer pink inside and the juices run clear. Remove the cutlets from the pan and set aside.

3. In a small bowl, whisk together the remaining 1 tablespoon oil and the vinegar.

4. Peel the hard-boiled eggs and slice each in half. Chop the cooked turkey into bite-size (about ¾-inch) pieces.

5. Put the lettuce in a large bowl and top with the tomatoes, bell pepper, eggs, and turkey. Drizzle the dressing on top.

Per serving (1½ cups): Calories: 213; Protein: 22g; Total Fat: 13g; Saturated Fat: 3g; Total Carbohydrates: 4g; Fiber: 2g; Cholesterol: 224mg; Phosphorus: 230mg; Potassium: 319mg; Sodium: 142mg; Sugar: 3g

Beef Kofta

STAGE 5

Serves 4 / Prep time: 10 minutes **/ Cook time:** 20 minutes

Big, bold Middle Eastern flavors make this dish a winner every time. Kofta (or kefta) are easy to prepare, but offer a complex taste profile that will have you eagerly waiting to dig in and have you coming back for more. You can easily replace the beef in this recipe with ground lamb, another iron-rich protein choice with an earthier flavor.

1 cup parboiled rice

12 ounces 93% lean ground beef

1 small white onion, chopped

2 garlic cloves, minced

1 teaspoon freshly ground black pepper

1 teaspoon ground cumin

1 teaspoon dried oregano

½ cup cherry tomatoes, halved

1 cup sliced cucumber

1 tablespoon red wine vinegar

1½ teaspoons olive oil

Tzatziki Sauce (page 113)

1. Cook the rice as directed on the package. Set aside.

2. Preheat the oven to 450°F. Line a baking sheet with parchment paper.

3. In a medium bowl, combine the beef, onion, garlic, pepper, cumin, and oregano and gently knead together. Divide the meat mixture into eight portions and form them into oblong ovals.

4. Place the kofta on the prepared baking sheet and bake for 12 to 15 minutes, until the juices run clear and the inside is no longer pink.

5. In a small bowl, mix together the tomatoes, cucumber, vinegar, and oil.

6. Serve the kofta alongside the salad and rice, with the tzatziki for dipping.

Per serving (2 kofta): Calories: 274; Protein: 22g; Total Fat: 6g; Saturated Fat: 2g; Total Carbohydrates: 32g; Fiber: 2g; Cholesterol: 53mg; Phosphorus: 214mg; Potassium: 451mg; Sodium: 62mg; Sugar: 2g

Pineapple BBQ Meatballs

STAGE 5

Serves 4 / Prep time: 15 minutes / **Cook time:** 25 minutes

These meatballs are great for entertaining—or just for you and your loved one! By hiding extra vegetables such as carrots in the meat mixture and pineapple in the sauce, you won't know you're eating something healthy. Serve these with rice or steamed vegetables to make a complete meal.

12 ounces 93% lean
    ground beef

1 tablespoon garlic powder

1 tablespoon onion powder

¼ cup rolled
    (old-fashioned) oats

½ cup shredded carrot

1 large egg

¼ cup BBQ Sauce
    (page 116)

1 (8-ounce) can pineapple
    tidbits in 100%
    juice, drained

1. Preheat the oven to 375°F. Line a baking sheet with parchment paper.

2. In a large bowl, combine the beef, garlic powder, onion powder, oats, carrot, and egg and mix well. Shape the mixture into 1-inch balls (you should have 24) and arrange them on the prepared baking sheet, spacing them evenly. Bake for 15 to 18 minutes, until no longer pink inside.

3. In a small saucepan, combine the BBQ sauce and pineapple. Simmer over medium heat for 3 to 5 minutes, or until the outside is brown and the juices run clear.

4. Transfer the meatballs to a large bowl, pour over the sauce, and toss until completely covered. Serve warm.

Per serving (6 meatballs): Calories: 212; Protein: 22g; Total Fat: 6g; Saturated Fat: 2g; Total Carbohydrates: 20g; Fiber: 2g; Cholesterol: 99mg; Phosphorus: 242mg; Potassium: 484mg; Sodium: 270mg; Sugar: 13g

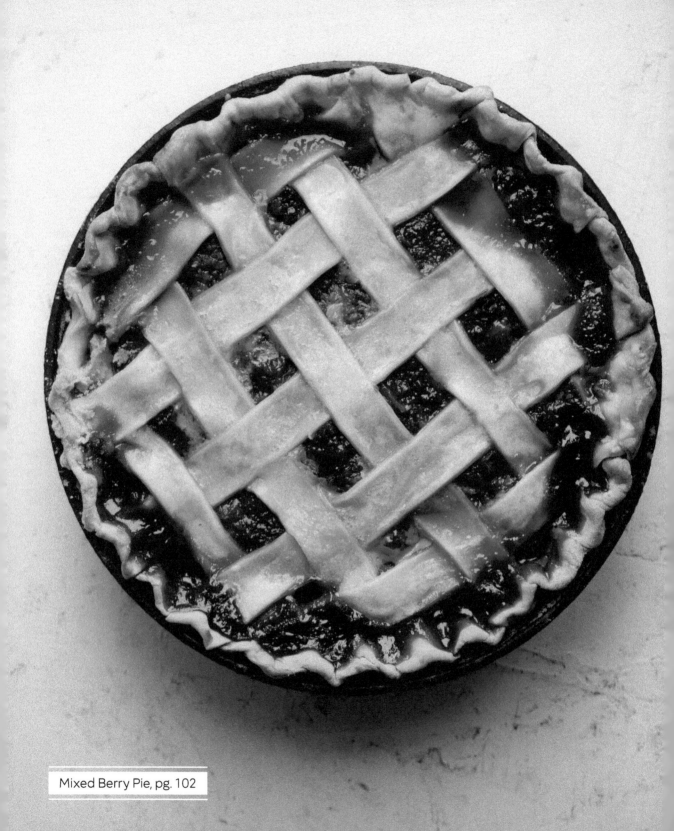

Mixed Berry Pie, pg. 102

Desserts

Peach-Blueberry Crumble

STAGES 1–3

*Serves 4 / **Prep time:** 5 minutes / **Cook time:** 30 minutes*

A crumble is a sweet dish that typically features stewed fruit and a crisp topping and is traditionally served with whipped cream. This peach-and-blueberry crumble is a perfect way to use up fresh fruit in the summer or frozen fruit in the winter (see Tip). If you don't have individual ramekins, you can use a muffin tin or a small cake pan; these may need a shorter cooking time, so be sure to watch closely as they bake.

Nonstick cooking spray

3 fresh peaches, pitted
and diced

1 cup fresh blueberries

1 teaspoon plus ¼ cup sugar

1 teaspoon lemon juice

½ cup rolled
(old-fashioned) oats

1 tablespoon
all-purpose flour

2 tablespoons unsalted
butter, melted

1 teaspoon ground
cinnamon

1. Preheat the oven to 375°F. Coat four oven-safe, 7-ounce ramekins with nonstick spray and set them on a baking sheet.

2. In a small bowl, combine the peaches, blueberries, 1 teaspoon of the sugar, and the lemon juice. Divide the fruit mixture evenly among the ramekins.

3. In a medium bowl, combine the oats, flour, remaining ¼ cup sugar, the melted butter, and the cinnamon. Spoon the crumble mixture evenly over the fruit in the ramekins.

4. Bake for 25 to 30 minutes, until the topping is golden brown and the fruit is bubbling.

TIP: You can use frozen fruit instead of fresh; just toss the fruit with 1 tablespoon cornstarch before adding the sugar and lemon juice (this helps to thicken the fruit sauce) and increase the baking time to 45 to 60 minutes.

Per serving (1 ramekin): Calories: 221; Protein: 4g; Total Fat: 7g; Saturated Fat: 4g; Total Carbohydrates: 39g; Fiber: 4g; Cholesterol: 15mg; Phosphorus: 95mg; Potassium: 309mg; Sodium: 2mg; Sugar: 26g

Dessert Pizza

STAGES 1–3

Serves 8 / Prep time: 15 minutes **/ Cook time:** 15 minutes

This dessert pizza is a fun homemade version of one you may get from your local pizza spot. Yes, it's a buttery, decadent dessert, but it's also a flavorful and sweet way to sneak some fresh fruit into your diet.

Nonstick cooking spray

¼ cup all-purpose flour, plus more for dusting

Pizza Dough (page 118)

2 tablespoons unsalted butter, at room temperature

⅓ cup sugar

2 tablespoons ground cinnamon

½ cup fresh blueberries

½ cup fresh raspberries

1. Preheat the oven to 450°F. Coat two large baking sheets with nonstick spray.

2. On a lightly floured counter, using your hands or a rolling pin, work each dough ball into a round. Place one round of dough on each prepared baking sheet.

3. In a small bowl, mix together the butter, flour, sugar, and cinnamon. Spread half of the mixture evenly over each dough round.

4. Bake the pizza crusts for 8 to 12 minutes, until golden brown.

5. While the pizzas are still warm, divide the fresh berries evenly between them, cut each into four slices, and enjoy.

Per serving (1 slice): Calories: 147; Protein: 3g; Total Fat: 3g; Saturated Fat: 2g; Total Carbohydrates: 27g; Fiber: 2g; Cholesterol: 8mg; Phosphorus: 29mg; Potassium: 50mg; Sodium: 94mg; Sugar: 10g

Mixed Berry Pie

STAGES 1–3

Serves 8 / Prep time: 10 minutes / **Cook time:** 55 minutes

This pie uses frozen berries, so you can enjoy the flavor of summer fruit all year long. Frozen fruit is a nutritious option and can be less expensive than fresh, but make sure to look for berries without any added sugar so the pie doesn't taste too sweet.

Pie Crust (page 119)
1½ cups frozen blackberries
1 cup frozen blueberries
1 cup frozen raspberries
1 cup sugar
⅓ cup cornstarch
1 tablespoon ground
   cinnamon

1. Preheat the oven to 375°F.

2. Combine the blackberries, blueberries, and rasp-berries in a microwave-safe medium bowl. On low power, thaw the berries in the microwave for 3 to 5 minutes. Watch closely so the berries do not burst. (Alternatively, let the berries thaw on the counter for 20 minutes.)

3. In a small bowl, mix together the sugar, cornstarch, and cinnamon. Add the sugar mixture to the bowl with the thawed berries and mix well.

4. On a floured surface, roll out one round of the pie dough, then transfer it to a 9-inch pie plate. Pour in the berry filling and spread it evenly.

5. Roll out the remaining round of dough and place it over the filling, then pinch the edges together to seal. Cut slits in the top crust. (Alternatively, make a lattice crust by cutting the dough into strips and weaving them in a crosshatch pattern over the filling.)

6. Bake the pie for 45 to 55 minutes, until the crust is golden brown and the juices are bubbling. Let cool on a wire rack for a few minutes before serving.

Per serving (1 slice): Calories: 432; Protein: 4g; Total Fat: 16g; Saturated Fat: 10g; Total Carbohydrates: 71g; Fiber: 5g; Cholesterol: 41mg; Phosphorus: 55mg; Potassium: 129mg; Sodium: 3mg; Sugar: 37g

Lemon Pie

STAGES 1–3

Serves 8 / Prep time: 10 minutes / **Cook time:** 40 minutes, plus 30 minutes cooling time

This lemon pie has a tart-and-sweet filling that will make your taste buds pop. The recipe calls for a homemade crust, but the filling is also delicious in a graham cracker crust, which you can purchase premade.

½ recipe Pie Crust (page 119)

1 cup lemon juice (from 3 or 4 lemons)

1 (14-ounce) can sweetened condensed milk

3 large egg yolks

1. Preheat the oven to 425°F.

2. Roll out the one round of the pie dough and transfer it to a 9-inch pie plate. Poke holes in the dough with a fork and bake for 20 minutes. Remove the pie crust from the oven and set aside to cool. Reduce the oven temperature to 375°F.

3. In a medium bowl, using a handheld mixer, beat the lemon juice, condensed milk, and egg yolks for 4 to 6 minutes, until the mixture reaches a smooth and cohesive consistency. Pour the filling into the cooled pie crust.

4. Bake the pie for 10 to 15 minutes, until the crust is brown and little bubbles have formed on the surface of the filling. Let cool on a wire rack in the refrigerator for 30 minutes before serving.

TIP: When separating the eggs for this recipe, reserve the egg whites to use in an omelet or a meringue topping. Store them in an airtight container in the refrigerator for up to 2 days or place them in a zip-top bag and freeze for up to 3 months.

Per serving (1 slice): Calories: 439; Protein: 9g; Total Fat: 21g; Saturated Fat: 13g; Total Carbohydrates: 54g; Fiber: 1g; Cholesterol: 127mg; Phosphorus: 191mg; Potassium: 260mg; Sodium: 69mg; Sugar: 29g

Chewy Chocolate Chip Cookies

STAGES 1–3

Makes 24 cookies / Prep time: 10 minutes / **Cook time:** 10 minutes

There is something so pure and perfect about a chewy chocolate chip cookie. These soft cookies are a breeze to prepare because they use melted butter, so you only need one bowl when mixing.

2½ cups all-purpose flour

1 teaspoon baking soda

1 tablespoon cornstarch

1 tablespoon vanilla extract

¾ cup (1½ sticks) unsalted butter, melted

1 cup sugar

2 large eggs

1 teaspoon ground cinnamon

½ cup mini dark chocolate chips

1. Preheat the oven to 325°F. Line a baking sheet with parchment paper.

2. In a medium bowl, using a handheld mixer, combine the flour, baking soda, cornstarch, vanilla, melted butter, sugar, eggs, and cinnamon and beat until well mixed. Stir in the chocolate chips with a wooden spoon or spatula.

3. Shape the dough into ½-inch balls, using about 2 tablespoons of dough for each, and place them about 2½ inches apart on the prepared baking sheet.

4. Bake for 10 minutes, or until the cookies are light brown and slightly puffed. Let cool on the baking sheet for about 2 minutes, then transfer to a wire rack to cool completely.

TIP: Add some extra protein to this recipe by stirring in ¼ cup chopped unsalted nuts with the chocolate chips in step 2.

Per serving (2 cookies): Calories: 316; Protein: 4g; Total Fat: 15g; Saturated Fat: 9g; Total Carbohydrates: 41g; Fiber: 1g; Cholesterol: 58mg; Phosphorus: 64mg; Potassium: 82mg; Sodium: 118mg; Sugar: 19g

Chocolate Bean Brownies

STAGES 1–3

Makes 12 brownies / Prep time: 10 minutes /
Cook time: 30 minutes, plus 30 minutes cooling time

These deep, rich, fudgy brownies are a healthier alternative to traditional brownies, and you'd never know they're made with black beans. Bonus: The beans serve up some extra fiber!

Nonstick cooking spray

1 (15-ounce) can
no-added-salt black
beans, drained and rinsed

2 tablespoons olive oil

3 large eggs

½ cup sugar

¼ cup unsweetened
cocoa powder

2 teaspoons vanilla extract

½ teaspoon cream of tartar

½ cup mini dark choco-
late chips

1. Preheat the oven to 350°F. Coat a 9-inch square baking pan with nonstick spray.

2. In a food processor, combine the black beans and oil and process until well blended. Add the eggs, sugar, cocoa powder, vanilla, and cream of tartar and process until well combined.

3. Transfer the batter to the prepared baking pan. Top the batter with the chocolate chips.

4. Bake for 25 to 30 minutes, until a toothpick inserted into the center comes out clean.

5. Let the brownies cool completely in the pan on a wire rack, about 30 minutes, then cut into 12 squares and serve.

TIP: Stored in an airtight container at room temperature, the brownies will stay fresh for 2 to 3 days. For longer storage, you can wrap each brownie individually in plastic wrap, place in an airtight container or zip-top bag, and freeze for 1 month.

Per serving (1 brownie): Calories: 143; Protein: 4g; Total Fat: 6g; Saturated Fat: 2g; Total Carbohydrates: 18g; Fiber: 3g; Cholesterol: 47mg; Phosphorus: 85mg; Potassium: 198mg; Sodium: 19mg; Sugar: 11g

Carrot Oatmeal Cookies

STAGES 1–3

Makes 24 cookies / **Prep time:** 10 minutes / **Cook time:** 20 minutes

These cookies are loaded with nutritious fruits and vegetables that provide more fiber and antioxidants than you'll find in a typical dessert. They make a great on-the-go snack or breakfast and taste just like carrot cake.

1 cup rolled
  (old-fashioned) oats
1 cup all-purpose flour
⅓ cup sugar
2 teaspoons ground
  cinnamon
1 teaspoon cream of tartar
1 tablespoon olive oil
1 cup grated carrots
½ cup grated apple
½ cup raisins

1. Preheat the oven to 375°F. Line a baking sheet with parchment paper.

2. In a medium bowl, using a handheld mixer, combine the oats, flour, sugar, cinnamon, cream of tartar, and oil. Fold in the carrots, apples, and raisins using a wooden spoon or spatula.

3. Shape the dough into ½-inch balls, using about 2 tablespoons of dough for each, and place them about 2½ inches apart on the prepared baking sheet. Using the palm of your hand, flatten the cookies to about ½ inch thick.

4. Bake for 18 to 20 minutes, until light brown and slightly puffed. Let the cookies cool on the baking sheet for about 2 minutes, then transfer to a wire rack to cool completely.

TIP: For those living with diabetes, swap out the sugar for ¼ cup unsweetened applesauce for a cookie that still tastes sweet without the refined sugar.

Per serving (2 cookies): Calories: 127; Protein: 3g; Total Fat: 2g; Saturated Fat: 0g; Total Carbohydrates: 26g; Fiber: 2g; Cholesterol: 0mg; Phosphorus: 64mg; Potassium: 169mg; Sodium: 8mg; Sugar: 10g

Raspberry-Lemon Bars

STAGE 4

Makes 12 bars / Prep time: 10 minutes / **Cook time:** 30 minutes, plus 30 minutes cooling time

These brightly colored raspberry-lemon bars come together in a snap and are packed with punchy citrus flavors. This recipe works well for a kidney-friendly diet because lemon and raspberries are low in potassium and phosphorus. These bars are a perfect summer dessert—no fork necessary!

Nonstick cooking spray

⅔ cup unsalted
    butter, melted

½ cup sugar

2 large eggs

2 tablespoons lemon juice

1 teaspoon vanilla extract

1½ cups all-purpose flour

1 cup fresh raspberries

1. Preheat the oven to 325°F. Coat an 8-inch square baking pan with nonstick spray.

2. In a large bowl, using a handheld mixer, combine the melted butter, sugar, eggs, lemon juice, and vanilla and beat until well mixed.

3. Stir in the flour until the batter is smooth. Fold in the raspberries with a spatula.

4. Pour the batter into the prepared pan. Bake for 30 minutes, or until golden on the edges. Let the bars cool completely in the pan on a wire rack, about 30 minutes, then cut into 12 squares and serve.

TIP: Stored in an airtight container at room temperature, the raspberry-lemon bars will stay fresh for 2 to 3 days (if they last that long!). For longer storage, wrap each bar individually in plastic wrap, place in an airtight container or zip-top bag, and freeze for up to 1 month.

Per serving (1 bar): Calories: 199; Protein: 3g; Total Fat: 11g; Saturated Fat: 7g; Total Carbohydrates: 22g; Fiber: 1g; Cholesterol: 58mg; Phosphorus: 40mg; Potassium: 50mg; Sodium: 14mg; Sugar: 9g

Snickerdoodle Cookies

STAGE 5

Makes 24 cookies / Prep time: 5 minutes / **Cook time:** 10 minutes

These cinnamon-y cookies are soft and chewy because of the cream of tartar. Often used as a baking powder substitute, cream of tartar in this recipe helps create the soft texture everyone loves in a butter-sugar cookie.

2 tablespoons sugar, plus 1 cup

3 tablespoons ground cinnamon

1 cup (2 sticks) unsalted butter, at room temperature

2 large eggs

1 tablespoon vanilla extract

3 cups all-purpose flour

2 teaspoons cream of tartar

1 teaspoon baking soda

1. Preheat the oven to 325°F. Line a baking sheet with parchment paper.

2. In a small bowl, mix together 2 tablespoons of the sugar and the cinnamon. Set aside.

3. In a medium bowl, using a handheld mixer, combine the remaining 1 cup sugar, the butter, eggs, vanilla, flour, cream of tartar, and baking soda and beat until well mixed.

4. Shape the dough into ½-inch balls, using about 2 tablespoons of dough for each, then roll them in the cinnamon-sugar mixture. Place the dough balls about 2½ inches apart on the prepared baking sheet and flatten them with a fork to prevent them from puffing up too much in the oven.

5. Bake the cookies for 10 minutes, or until light brown and slightly puffed. Let cool on the baking sheet for about 2 minutes, then transfer to a wire rack to cool completely.

Per serving (2 cookies): Calories: 348; Protein: 5g; Total Fat: 16g; Saturated Fat: 10g; Total Carbohydrates: 46g; Fiber: 2g; Cholesterol: 72mg; Phosphorus: 56mg; Potassium: 142mg; Sodium: 120mg; Sugar: 20g

Cinnamon Roll Cake

STAGE 5

Serves 12 / Prep time: 5 minutes / **Cook time:** 35 minutes

Easier to prepare than cinnamon rolls, this cake is packed with just as much flavor. It's a gooey and delicious dessert best served warm, right out of the oven.

Nonstick cooking spray

3 cups all-purpose flour

1 cup sugar

¼ teaspoon salt

4 teaspoons cream of tartar

1½ cups unsweetened plain almond milk

2 large eggs

1 tablespoon vanilla extract

½ cup (1 stick) unsalted butter, at room temperature, divided

½ cup ground cinnamon, divided

1. Preheat the oven to 325°F. Coat a 9-by-13-inch baking pan with nonstick spray.

2. In a large bowl, using a handheld mixer, combine the flour, sugar, salt, cream of tartar, almond milk, eggs, vanilla, 4 tablespoons (½ stick) of the butter, and ¼ cup of the cinnamon and beat until well mixed. Pour the batter into the prepared baking pan.

3. In a small bowl, mix together the remaining 4 tablespoons (½ stick) butter and ¼ cup cinnamon. Drop dollops of the cinnamon butter evenly throughout the cake batter and use a knife to create swirls (do not mix to combine).

4. Bake for 25 to 35 minutes, until the cake is golden brown on the edges and a toothpick inserted into the center comes out clean. Let the cake cool in the pan on a wire rack for a few minutes before slicing and serving.

TIP: To reheat the cake slices, preheat the oven to 350°F. Cover slices with aluminum foil and warm for about 10 minutes.

Per serving (1 slice): Calories: 287; Protein: 5g; Total Fat: 9g; Saturated Fat: 5g; Total Carbohydrates: 47g; Fiber: 4g; Cholesterol: 48mg; Phosphorus: 56mg; Potassium: 250mg; Sodium: 81mg; Sugar: 19g

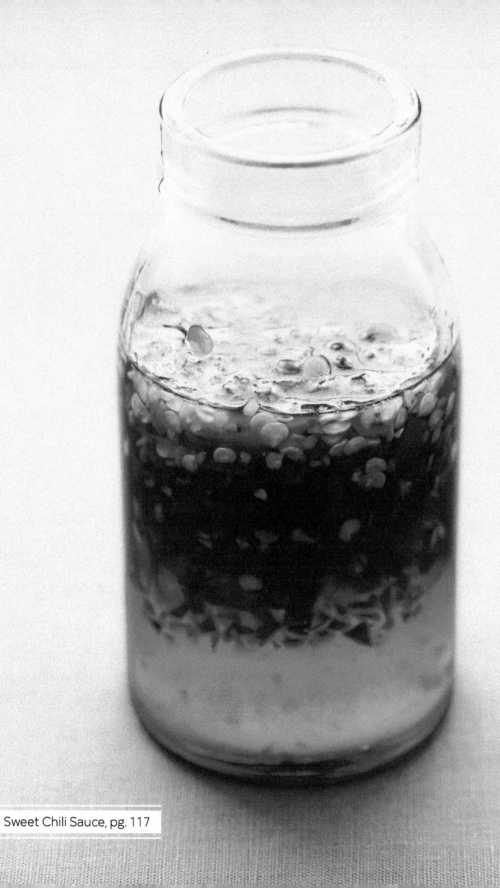

Sweet Chili Sauce, pg. 117

Homemade Staples

Tahini Sauce

Makes ½ cup / Prep time: 5 minutes

Tahini is a Middle Eastern condiment made of ground sesame seeds and is typically used to make hummus and baba ghanoush. This is a nutty, bitter, and savory tahini sauce you can add to any salad, bowl, or roasted vegetable dish.

2 tablespoons tahini

3 tablespoon warm water, plus more as needed

2 tablespoons lemon juice

1 tablespoon olive oil

2 garlic cloves, minced

1. In a medium bowl, whisk together the tahini and warm water until smooth.

2. Add the lemon juice, oil, and garlic, and whisk until creamy and smooth.

3. Use immediately or in an airtight container in the refrigerator for up to 2 days. The sauce will thicken up in the refrigerator; add warm water and stir until smooth before enjoying.

TIP: Adjust the lemon juice to taste or add red pepper flakes to kick up the flavor.

Per serving (¼ cup): Calories: 160; Protein: 3g; Total Fat: 15g; Saturated Fat: 2g; Total Carbohydrates: 5g; Fiber: 2g; Cholesterol: 0mg; Phosphorus: 120mg; Potassium: 92mg; Sodium: 19mg; Sugar: 0g

Tzatziki Sauce

Makes ½ cup / Prep time: 10 minutes

Tzatziki is a light, creamy, and flavorful condiment. It is great for topping salads, vegetables, and sandwiches, or to serve with pitas for dipping. You'll be amazed at how much flavor is packed in this simple recipe.

¼ cup low-fat plain Greek yogurt

1 tablespoon lemon juice

¼ teaspoon freshly ground black pepper

2 teaspoons dried dill

1 garlic clove, minced

1 cup finely diced cucumber

1. In a small bowl, combine the yogurt, lemon juice, pepper, dill, garlic, and cucumber and mix well.

2. Use immediately or store the tzatziki in an airtight container in the refrigerator for up to 3 days.

Per serving (2 tablespoons): Calories: 18; Protein: 1g; Total Fat: 1g; Saturated Fat: 0g; Total Carbohydrates: 3g; Fiber: 0g; Cholesterol: 2mg; Phosphorus: 25mg; Potassium: 81mg; Sodium: 8mg; Sugar: 0g

Pickled Vegetables

Makes 2 cups / Prep time: 10 minutes, plus 30 minutes cooling time

When a loved one must limit sodium because of their CKD, it often means we need to limit the extra toppings or condiments on our foods. These low-sodium pickled vegetables are a great way to add some extra flavor, color, and crunch to your meal without all the added salt.

2 cups very thinly sliced vegetables (carrots, radishes, red onion, cauliflower)

1 cup water

¾ cup apple cider vinegar

1 tablespoon sugar

1 teaspoon salt

1. Put the vegetables into a 1-pint Mason jar.

2. In a small saucepan, combine the water, vinegar, sugar, and salt and bring to a boil over high heat, stirring to dissolve the sugar and salt.

3. Pour the hot liquid into the jar so that all the vegetables are submerged. Cover with the lid and let cool to room temperature, about 30 minutes. Enjoy immediately or store in the refrigerator for 1 to 2 months (because these quick pickles have not been processed by canning, they cannot be stored at room temperature).

TIP: Use other vegetables, like beets, green beans, zucchini, or bell peppers, when they're in season, and flavor the pickling liquid with red pepper flakes, garlic cloves, or fresh dill.

Per serving (½ cup): Calories: 81; Protein: 3g; Total Fat: 0g; Saturated Fat: 0g; Total Carbohydrates: 15g; Fiber: 4g; Cholesterol: 0mg; Phosphorus: 50mg; Potassium: 187mg; Sodium: 423mg; Sugar: 6g

Spicy Sauce

Makes ½ cup / Prep time: 5 minutes

Because this recipe uses Greek yogurt as a base, the result is a creamy sauce packed with lots of spice. Serve it with salads or bowls, or try using it as a dip for vegetables.

½ cup low-fat plain
  Greek yogurt
1 teaspoon paprika
1 teaspoon ground cumin
¼ teaspoon garlic powder
¼ teaspoon onion powder
¼ teaspoon red
  pepper flakes

1. In a small bowl, stir together the yogurt, paprika, cumin, garlic powder, onion powder, and red pepper flakes until well combined.

2. Use immediately or in an airtight container in the refrigerator for up to 3 days.

Per serving (2 tablespoons): Calories: 24; Protein: 1g; Total Fat: 1g; Saturated Fat: 1g; Total Carbohydrates: 2g; Fiber: 1g; Cholesterol: 4mg; Phosphorus: 35mg; Potassium: 75mg; Sodium: 16mg; Sugar: 2g

BBQ Sauce

Makes ½ cup / Prep time: 5 minutes / **Cook time:** 5 minutes, plus 20 minutes cooling time

This homemade BBQ Sauce is low in sodium, making it a great option for topping meats like beef or chicken. Barbecue sauce is typically high in potassium and sodium because it is made with ketchup.

4 ounces low-sodium
tomato sauce

1 tablespoon apple
cider vinegar

1 tablespoon sugar

1 teaspoon paprika

½ teaspoon garlic powder

½ teaspoon onion powder

1. In a small saucepan, combine the tomato sauce, vinegar, sugar, paprika, garlic powder, and onion powder. Bring to a gentle simmer over medium-high heat, stirring often, and cook for 5 minutes.

2. Remove from the heat and let cool in the refrigerator for 15 to 20 minutes before enjoying. Store in an airtight container in the refrigerator for up to 1 week.

Per serving (2 tablespoons): Calories: 24; Protein: 1g; Total Fat: 0g; Saturated Fat: 0g; Total Carbohydrates: 6g; Fiber: 1g; Cholesterol: 0mg; Phosphorus: 12mg; Potassium: 108mg; Sodium: 4mg; Sugar: 4g

Sweet Chili Sauce

Makes ¼ cup / Prep time: 5 minutes **/ Cook time:** 5 minutes, plus 30 minutes cooling time

Sweet chili sauce is a sweet-and-spicy condiment popular in Thailand. This homemade option omits the fish sauce found in the traditional version, making it a low-sodium option.

2 tablespoons water

⅛ teaspoon cornstarch

1 small fresh serrano chile, finely chopped

¼ cup apple cider vinegar

½ cup sugar

1 garlic clove, minced

1 teaspoon minced fresh ginger

1. In a small bowl, combine the water and cornstarch to make a paste.

2. In a small saucepan, combine the serrano, vinegar, sugar, garlic, and ginger and bring to a boil. Reduce the heat, stir in the cornstarch paste, and simmer for 2 minutes.

3. Remove from the heat and let cool for 30 minutes at room temperature before serving. Store in an airtight container in the refrigerator for up to 1 month.

TIP: Remove the seeds from the serrano chile to reduce the heat.

Per serving (¾ teaspoon): Calories: 26; Protein: 0g; Total Fat: 0g; Saturated Fat: 0g; Total Carbohydrates: 6g; Fiber: 0g; Cholesterol: 0mg; Phosphorus: 1mg; Potassium: 5mg; Sodium: 0mg; Sugar: 6g

Pizza Dough

Makes dough for 2 pizzas (to serve 4) / **Prep time:** 20 minutes

This pizza dough is quick and easy, with none of the phosphate additives you'll find in many store-bought options. Whether you finish it with savory or sweet toppings, it won't disappoint.

1 cup warm water

1 teaspoon instant yeast

1 teaspoon sugar

2 cups all-purpose flour, plus more for dusting

½ teaspoon salt

1. In a medium bowl, combine the water, yeast, and sugar. Let stand until foamy, about 5 minutes.

2. Add the flour and salt to the yeast mixture and stir until it forms a ball.

3. Turn the dough out onto a lightly floured surface and knead for about 10 minutes, until smooth. Form the dough into a ball and let it rest for 5 minutes.

4. Divide the dough in half and form each portion into a ball. Use as directed in your pizza recipe or wrap each ball in plastic wrap and store in the refrigerator for up to 48 hours. For longer storage, place the wrapped dough in a zip-top bag and freeze for up to 3 months. Let frozen dough defrost on the counter for 2 hours before using; it should be pliable, but still firm in texture.

TIP: To make your pizzas, unwrap the dough on a floured countertop and, using your hands or a rolling pin, flatten each ball into a round.

Per serving (½ pizza, crust only): Calories: 235; Protein: 7g; Total Fat: 1g; Saturated Fat: 1g; Total Carbohydrates: 49g; Fiber: 2g; Cholesterol: 0mg; Phosphorus: 74mg; Potassium: 77mg; Sodium: 294mg; Sugar: 1g

Pie Crust

Makes dough for 1 double-crust pie / Prep time: 10 minutes

The basics of a pie crust are flour, fat, and water, so making your own dough should not be intimidating. This recipe breaks it down so you can create that buttery, flavorful pie crust everyone loves right in your own kitchen.

2 cups all-purpose flour, plus more for dusting

1½ teaspoons sugar

⅔ cup unsalted butter, cut into ¼-inch pieces and chilled

5 tablespoons cold water

1. In a food processor, combine the flour, sugar, and cold butter and pulse until the mixture becomes dry, coarse, and crumbly.

2. Add the water 1 tablespoon at a time and pulse until a small ball of dough forms.

3. Transfer the dough from the food processor to a lightly floured surface and knead for 2 to 4 minutes, until smooth.

4. Divide the dough into two portions, form each into a ball, and wrap in plastic wrap. Chill in the refrigerator for at least 5 minutes or up to 3 days before using, or place the wrapped dough in a zip-top bag and freeze for up to 3 months. Thaw frozen dough in the refrigerator overnight or let stand at room temperature until pliable but firm before rolling it out.

Per serving (⅛ recipe): Calories: 253; Protein: 3g; Total Fat: 16g; Saturated Fat: 10g; Total Carbohydrates: 25g; Fiber: 1g; Cholesterol: 41mg; Phosphorus: 38mg; Potassium: 38mg; Sodium: 3mg; Sugar: 1g

Spice Mixes

Preparing homemade spice mixes is a great way to add flavor to your foods without adding sodium. Store each mix in an airtight container with a tight-fitting lid in a cool, dark place for up to 6 months.

Greek Seasoning

Makes 2½ tablespoons

Swap out the oregano and dill in the Greek Chickpea Power Bowl (page 60) for this seasoning for an extra punch of Mediterranean flavor.

2 teaspoons ground cumin
2 teaspoons paprika
1 teaspoon garlic powder
1 teaspoon onion powder
½ teaspoon dried dill
1 teaspoon dried oregano

In a small bowl, mix together the cumin, paprika, garlic powder, onion powder, dill, and oregano.

Per serving (about 2 teaspoons): Calories: 27; Protein: 1g; Total Fat: 1g; Saturated Fat: 0g; Total Carbohydrates: 5g; Fiber: 2g; Cholesterol: 0mg; Phosphorus: 30mg; Potassium: 133mg; Sodium: 7mg; Sugar: 0g

Mexican Seasoning

Makes 2 teaspoons

Add this seasoning to Black Bean Burgers (page 57) to give them a punchier flavor profile.

½ teaspoon paprika
½ teaspoon ground cumin
¼ teaspoon garlic powder
¼ teaspoon onion powder
¼ teaspoon red pepper flakes
¼ teaspoon dried oregano

In a small bowl, mix together the paprika, cumin, garlic powder, onion powder, red pepper flakes, and oregano.

Per serving (¼ teaspoon): Calories: 2; Protein: 0g; Total Fat: 0g; Saturated Fat: 0g; Total Carbohydrates: 0g; Fiber: 0g; Cholesterol: 0mg; Phosphorus: 2mg; Potassium: 10mg; Sodium: 0mg; Sugar: 0g

Italian Blend Seasoning

Makes 5 teaspoons

Instead of using oregano in the High-Protein Shakshuka recipe (page 49), go with this spice blend for a more intense flavor.

1½ teaspoons dried oregano
1½ teaspoons dried parsley
1 teaspoon red pepper flakes
1 teaspoon garlic powder

In a small bowl, mix together the oregano, parsley, red pepper flakes, and garlic powder.

Per serving (1¼ teaspoons): Calories: 5; Protein: 0g; Total Fat: 0g; Saturated Fat: 0g; Total Carbohydrates: 1g; Fiber: 0g; Cholesterol: 0mg; Phosphorus: 5mg; Potassium: 26mg; Sodium: 1mg; Sugar: 0g

Everything Bagel Seasoning

Makes 1 tablespoon

Add this seasoning to Tzatziki Egg Salad (page 63) for an egg salad sandwich with a twist.

1 teaspoon dried
  minced onion
1 teaspoon dried
  minced garlic
½ teaspoon sesame seeds
¼ teaspoon red
  pepper flakes
¼ teaspoon poppy seeds

In a small bowl, mix together the dried onion, dried garlic, sesame seeds, red pepper flakes, and poppy seeds.

Per serving (¾ teaspoon): Calories: 6; Protein: 0g; Total Fat: 0g; Saturated Fat: 0g; Total Carbohydrates: 1g; Fiber: 0g; Cholesterol: 0mg; Phosphorus: 7mg; Potassium: 15mg; Sodium: 1mg; Sugar: 0g

Cinnamon Sugar

Makes 4 teaspoons

For a sweet midafternoon snack, add this classic mix to plain yogurt and serve it with fruit for dipping. Or sprinkle some on top of the Cinnamon Roll Cake (page 109) for an extra-sweet crust.

1 tablespoon ground
  cinnamon
1 teaspoon sugar

In a small bowl, mix together the cinnamon and sugar.

Per serving (1 teaspoon): Calories: 9; Protein: 0g; Total Fat: 0g; Saturated Fat: 0g; Total Carbohydrates: 2g; Fiber: 1g; Cholesterol: 0mg; Phosphorus: 1mg; Potassium: 8mg; Sodium: 0mg; Sugar: 1g

Food Lists for the Renal Diet

Potassium

HIGHER-POTASSIUM LEGUMES*
Greater than 300mg per cooked ½-cup serving

- Pinto beans
- Lentils
- Kidney beans
- Black beans

LOWER-POTASSIUM LEGUMES
Less than 300mg per serving specified

- ¼ cup chopped peanuts
- 4 ounces tofu
- ½ cup chickpeas
- 2 tablespoons peanut butter

HIGHER-POTASSIUM NUTS
Greater than 200mg per ¼-cup serving

- Pistachios (shelled)
- Brazil nuts
- Cashews
- Pine nuts
- Almonds

LOWER-POTASSIUM NUTS
Less than 200mg per ¼-cup serving

- Pecans
- Walnuts
- Macadamia nuts

HIGHER-POTASSIUM SEAFOOD
Greater than 300mg per cooked 3-ounce serving (unless otherwise specified)

- Salmon
- Trout
- Sardines
- Atlantic mackerel
- Tilapia
- 4 clams
- 4 raw oysters

LOWER-POTASSIUM SEAFOOD

Less than 300mg per cooked 3-ounce serving

- Cod
- Sea bass
- Scallops
- Shrimp
- Crab
- Lobster
- Sole
- Flounder

HIGHER-POTASSIUM MEAT, POULTRY, AND EGGS

Greater than 300mg per cooked 3-ounce serving

- Pork chop
- Pork tenderloin
- Steak

LOWER-POTASSIUM MEAT, POULTRY, AND EGGS

Less than 300mg per cooked 3-ounce serving (unless otherwise specified)

- Veal
- Lamb
- Ground beef
- Turkey breast
- Chicken breast
- Chicken thigh
- 3 large egg whites
- 2 large eggs

HIGHER-POTASSIUM DAIRY AND DAIRY-ALTERNATIVE FOODS

Greater than 300mg per serving specified

- 1 cup evaporated milk
- 1 cup low-fat milk
- 5-ounce container low-fat plain yogurt
- 1 cup whole milk
- 1 cup soy milk

LOWER-POTASSIUM DAIRY AND DAIRY-ALTERNATIVE FOODS

Less than 300mg per serving specified

- 5-ounce container low-fat plain Greek yogurt
- 5-ounce container full-fat plain yogurt
- 1 cup unenriched rice milk
- 5-ounce container full-fat plain Greek yogurt
- 5 ounces plain almond-milk yogurt
- 5 ounces cottage cheese
- ½ cup chocolate ice cream
- 1 cup almond milk
- ½ cup vanilla ice cream
- 1 ounce cheese (most types)

HIGHER-POTASSIUM GRAINS AND STARCHES**

Greater than 200mg per cooked 1-cup serving (unless otherwise specified)

- 1 medium white potato, peeled and boiled
- 1 medium sweet potato, peeled and boiled
- Quinoa

LOWER-POTASSIUM GRAINS AND STARCHES

Less than 200mg per cooked 1-cup serving (unless otherwise specified)

- Steel-cut oats
- 2 medium whole wheat bread slices
- Bulgur
- Peas
- Brown rice
- Wild rice
- Pearled barley
- Rolled (old-fashioned) oats
- 1 whole wheat English muffin
- Whole wheat spaghetti
- Polenta
- 2 medium rye bread slices
- Couscous
- Spaghetti
- White rice

LOWER-POTASSIUM FRUITS

Less than 200mg per ½ cup fresh or canned, or 1 small whole fruit (unless otherwise specified)

- Apple
- Applesauce
- Apricot (fresh)
- Berries
- Cherries
- Clementine
- Dried apples, blueberries, cherries, or cranberries (¼ cup)
- Fruit cup (any fruit), fruit cocktail
- Grapes
- Lemon or lime
- Pear
- Pineapple
- Plum
- Tangerine or mandarin orange
- Watermelon (1 cup)

HIGHER-POTASSIUM FRUITS

More than 200mg per ½ cup fresh or canned, or 1 small whole fruit (unless otherwise specified)

- Avocado
- Banana
- Dried fruit: raisins, dates, figs, apricots, bananas, peaches, pears, or prunes (¼ cup)
- Honeydew
- Kiwi
- Nectarine
- Orange
- Papaya
- Peach
- Plantain
- Pomegranate

LOWER-POTASSIUM VEGETABLES

Less than 200mg per 1 cup fresh leafy greens or ½ cup fresh, cooked, or canned vegetables

- Alfalfa sprouts
- Asparagus
- Bamboo shoots (canned)
- Bean sprouts
- Beets (canned)
- Broccoli
- Cabbage
- Carrots
- Cauliflower
- Celery
- Cucumber
- Eggplant
- Green or wax beans
- Greens: collard, mustard, or turnip
- Jicama/yam bean
- Lettuce: all types
- Mushrooms (raw or canned)
- Okra
- Onion or leek
- Peas: green, sugar snap, or snow peas
- Peppers: green, red, or yellow
- Radish
- Rhubarb
- Spinach (raw)
- Spaghetti squash
- Cherry tomatoes
- Turnip
- Yellow summer squash
- Water chestnuts (canned)

HIGHER-POTASSIUM VEGETABLES

More than 200mg per 1 cup leafy greens or ½ cup fresh, cooked, or canned vegetables (unless otherwise specified)*

- Acorn squash
- Artichoke
- Beet greens
- Brussels sprouts
- Butternut squash
- Chard, cooked
- Chinese cabbage, cooked
- Corn (1 ear)
- Edamame
- Hubbard squash
- Kohlrabi
- Lentils
- Parsnips**
- Potatoes**
- Pumpkins
- Rutabaga**
- Spinach, cooked
- Tomato
- Tomato sauce, tomato paste, and tomato juice
- Vegetable juice
- Yams**
- Zucchini

*These higher-potassium legumes can fit into a low-potassium diet as long as you stick to the serving size and avoid combining them with higher-potassium vegetables, grains, and/or meat, poultry, or fish.

**High-potassium root vegetables, such as potatoes, can be double boiled to reduce their potassium content. Simply peel and slice or dice your potatoes, boil for 15 minutes, and drain. Boil again in fresh water until tender and cooked to your liking.

Protein

Protein-rich foods include meat, poultry, fish, eggs, milk, cheese, legumes, nuts, and grains. Fruits and vegetables contain very low levels of protein and are therefore not included.

LEGUMES

Per cooked ½-cup serving (unless otherwise specified)

- Black beans 8g
- Chickpeas 7g
- Kidney beans 8g
- Lentils 9g
- Peanuts (¼ cup) 9g
- Peas 8g
- Pinto beans 8g
- Soybeans 16g
- Tofu, not silken, 15g; silken, 10g
- 2 tablespoons peanut butter 7g

NUTS

Per ¼-cup serving

- Almonds 7g
- Brazil nuts 5g
- Cashews 6g
- Macadamia nuts 2g
- Pecans 3g
- Pine nuts 4g
- Pistachios 6g
- Walnuts 5g

GRAINS AND STARCHES

Per cooked 1-cup serving (unless otherwise specified)

- Brown rice 6g
- Bulgur 6g
- Couscous 6g
- Pearled barley 5g
- Polenta/grits 4g
- Quinoa 8g
- Rolled (old-fashioned) oats 6g
- Rye bread (2 medium slices) 5g
- Steel-cut oats 7g
- White rice 4g
- Whole wheat bread (2 medium slices) 9g
- Whole wheat English muffin 6g
- Whole wheat or regular spaghetti 8g
- Wild rice 7g

SEAFOOD

Per cooked 3-ounce serving (unless otherwise specified)

- Atlantic mackerel 20g
- Clams (4) 12g
- Cod 17g
- Crab 15g
- Flounder 13g
- Lobster 16g
- Raw oysters (4) 17g
- Salmon 22g
- Sardines 22g
- Scallops 18g
- Sea bass 20g
- Shrimp 20g
- Sole 13g
- Tilapia 22g
- Trout 20g

MEAT, POULTRY, AND EGGS

Per cooked 3-ounce serving (unless otherwise specified)

- Chicken breast 26g
- Chicken thigh 24g
- Eggs (2 large) 13g
- Egg whites (3 large) 11g
- Ground beef 22g
- Lamb 24g
- Pork chop 25g
- Pork tenderloin 24g
- Steak 25g
- Turkey breast 26g
- Veal 21g

PROTEIN IN DAIRY AND DAIRY-ALTERNATIVE FOODS

Per 1-cup serving (unless otherwise specified)

- Almond milk 1g
- Almond-milk yogurt (5 ounces) 6g
- Cheese (most types, 1 ounce), 6g to 8g
- Evaporated milk 17g
- Full-fat plain yogurt (5 ounces) 5g
- Ice cream (½ cup) 3g
- Low-fat cottage cheese (5 ounces) 15g
- Low-fat milk 8g
- Low-fat plain Greek yogurt (5 ounces) 15g
- Low-fat plain Greek yogurt (5 ounces) 13g
- Low-fat plain yogurt (5 ounces) 7g
- Soy milk 8g
- Unenriched rice milk 2g
- Whole milk 8g

Sodium

HIGH-SODIUM FOODS TO LIMIT

Check food labels for actual sodium content per serving

- Bacon
- Baking mixes (pancakes, desserts)
- Barbecue sauce
- Bouillon cubes
- Bread
- Buttermilk
- Canned ravioli
- Cold cuts, deli meat
- Corned beef
- Fast foods
- Frozen prepared foods
- Garlic salt
- Ham
- High-sodium cereals
- Hot dogs
- Ketchup
- Microwave meals
- Monosodium glutamate (MSG)
- Most canned foods (unless specified as no-added-salt or low-sodium)
- Onion salt
- Potato chips
- Salad dressings
- Salted crackers
- Sauerkraut
- Sausage
- Seasoning salt
- Smoked fish
- Soy sauce
- Spam
- Steak sauce
- Table salt
- Teriyaki sauce
- Vegetable juices

LOW-SODIUM FOODS TO CHOOSE

Check food labels for actual sodium content per serving

- Allspice
- Black pepper
- Canned food with no added salt
- Crackers, unsalted
- Dill
- Dry mustard
- Eggs
- Fresh fish
- Fresh garlic
- Fresh onion
- Ginger
- Homemade or no-added-salt broth
- Lemon juice
- Lower-sodium breads and cereals (check labels)
- Low-sodium salad dressings
- Low-sodium seasoning blends
- Nuts, unsalted
- Pretzels, unsalted
- Rosemary
- Sage
- Tarragon
- Thyme
- Unsalted popcorn
- Vinegar, regular or flavored

Phosphorus

Phosphorus is found in protein-rich foods. Fruits and vegetables contain very small amounts of phosphorus and are therefore not included. Tables include total phosphorus and phosphorus adjusted for estimated bioavailability in descending order.

Plant Sources of Phosphorus: Low Bioavailability

PHOSPHORUS IN LEGUMES

Per cooked ½-cup serving (unless otherwise specified)

FOOD	PHOSPHORUS	ADJUSTED PHOSPHORUS*
Soybeans	211mg	106mg
Lentils	178mg	89mg
Chickpeas	138mg	69mg
¼ cup peanuts	137mg	69mg
Pinto beans	126mg	63mg
Kidney beans	122mg	61mg
4 ounces tofu (not silken)	122mg	61mg
Black beans	120mg	60mg
2 tablespoons peanut butter	108mg	54mg
4 ounces silken tofu	102mg	51mg

*Adjusted phosphorus was calculated using an estimate of 50% bioavailability of phosphorus in plant sources.

PHOSPHORUS IN NUTS

Per ¼-cup serving

FOOD	PHOSPHORUS	ADJUSTED PHOSPHORUS*
Brazil nuts	241mg	121mg
Pine nuts	194mg	97mg
Cashews	191mg	96mg
Almonds	156mg	78mg
Pistachios	151mg	76mg
Walnuts	101mg	51mg
Pecans	76mg	38mg
Macadamia nuts	63mg	32mg

*Adjusted phosphorus was calculated using an estimate of 50% bioavailability of phosphorus in plant sources.

PHOSPHORUS IN GRAINS AND STARCHES
Per cooked 1-cup serving

FOOD	PHOSPHORUS	ADJUSTED PHOSPHORUS*
Quinoa	281mg	141mg
Steel-cut oats	219mg	110mg
Brown rice	208mg	104mg
Whole wheat spaghetti	178mg	89mg
Rolled (old-fashioned) oats	172mg	86mg
Wild rice	135mg	68mg
Bulgur	134mg	67mg
Pearled barley	121mg	61mg
Couscous	80mg	40mg
Polenta/grits	53mg	27mg

*Adjusted phosphorus was calculated using an estimate of 50% bioavailability of phosphorus in plant sources.

Animal Sources of Phosphorus: Medium Bioavailability

PHOSPHORUS IN SEAFOOD
Per cooked 3-ounce serving (unless otherwise specified)

FOOD	PHOSPHORUS	ADJUSTED PHOSPHORUS*
Scallops	362mg	253mg
4 raw oysters	294mg	206mg
Sardines	272mg	190mg
Sole	263mg	184mg
Flounder	262mg	183mg
Atlantic mackerel	236mg	165mg
Trout	230mg	161mg
Salmon	218mg	153mg
Sea bass	211mg	148mg
Shrimp	202mg	141mg
Crab	199mg	139mg
Tilapia	174mg	122mg
4 clams	164mg	115mg
Lobster	157mg	81mg
Light tuna	139mg	97mg
Cod	117mg	82mg

*Adjusted phosphorus was calculated using an estimate of 70% bioavailability of phosphorus in animal sources.

Phosphorus Cooking Tip: Research shows that preparing meats by boiling them in liquid can reduce their phosphorus content by 10 to 50 percent. This works best when the meat is sliced before cooking. Because the phosphorus is leached into the liquid, you'll need to discard the cooking liquid before serving.

PHOSPHORUS IN MEAT, POULTRY, AND EGGS

Per cooked 3-ounce serving (unless otherwise specified)

FOOD	PHOSPHORUS	ADJUSTED PHOSPHORUS*
Pork tenderloin	248mg	174mg
Steak	230mg	161mg
Turkey breast	196mg	137mg
Veal	190mg	133mg
Pork chop	189mg	132mg
Chicken breast	184mg	129mg
Chicken thigh	180mg	126mg
Lamb	173mg	121mg
Ground beef	158mg	111mg
2 large eggs	172mg	120mg
Hamburger	158mg	111mg
3 large egg whites	15mg	11mg

*Adjusted phosphorus was calculated using an estimate of 70% bioavailability of phosphorus in animal sources.

PHOSPHORUS IN DAIRY FOODS

FOOD	PHOSPHORUS	ADJUSTED PHOSPHORUS*
1 cup evaporated milk	460mg	322mg
1 cup low-fat milk	225mg	158mg
5 ounces low-fat cottage cheese	213mg	149mg
1 cup whole milk	205mg	144mg
5-ounce container low-fat plain yogurt	204mg	143mg
5-ounce container full-fat plain Greek yogurt	191mg	134mg
5-ounce container low-fat plain Greek yogurt	141mg	99mg
5-ounce container full-fat plain yogurt	135mg	95mg
1 ounce cheese (most types)	130 to 180mg	91 to 126mg
1 ounce feta cheese	96mg	67mg
1 ounce goat cheese	73mg	51mg
½ cup ice cream	69mg	48mg
1 ounce Brie cheese	53mg	37mg

*Adjusted phosphorus was calculated using an estimate of 70% bioavailability of phosphorus in animal sources.

Processed Sources of Phosphorus: High Bioavailability (80 to 100%)

The food industry is not required to provide the phosphorus content of processed foods. Foods with phosphorus additives represent the most bioavailable form of phosphorus in the diet. The following foods frequently contain phosphorus additives. Always check the ingredient label to be sure.

- Fast food ("fast-fresh" food may be okay)
- Bottled drinks such as soda, flavored waters, juices
- Certain brands of nondairy creamers or half-and-half
- Certain brands of nondairy milks

- Processed meats (includes all cold cuts, as well as breakfast meats such as sausage, bacon, and turkey bacon)
- Frozen prepared meals
- Many canned foods
- Processed sweet and savory snack foods (cakes, cookies, cheese-based snacks)

High-Fiber Carbohydrates

Fiber is found in vegetables, fruits, whole grains, nuts, and legumes.

HIGH-FIBER LEGUMES

Per cooked ½-cup serving

- Black beans 8g
- Chickpeas 5g
- Kidney beans 6g

- Lentils 6g
- Peas 7g
- Pinto beans 8g

HIGH-FIBER NUTS

Per ¼-cup serving

- Almonds 4g
- Brazil nuts 3g
- Macadamia nuts 3g

- Pecans 3g
- Pistachios 3g

HIGH-FIBER GRAINS AND STARCHES

Per cooked 1-cup serving (unless otherwise specified)

- Brown rice 3g
- Bulgur 6g
- Quinoa 5g
- Rolled (old-fashioned) oats 8g
- 2 medium rye bread slices 3g
- 2 medium whole wheat bread slices 4g
- Steel-cut oats 5g
- 1 medium sweet potato 4g
- 1 medium white potato 4g
- 1 whole wheat English muffin 4g
- Whole wheat spaghetti 6g

HIGH-FIBER FRUITS

Per ½ cup fresh or canned, or 1 small whole fruit (unless otherwise specified)

- Apple 4g
- ¼ avocado 2g
- Blackberries 4g
- Blueberries 2g
- Mandarin orange 2g
- Pear 6g
- Raspberries 4g
- Strawberries 2g

HIGH-FIBER VEGETABLES

Per cooked ½-cup serving (unless otherwise specified)

- Asparagus 2g
- Broccoli 3g
- Brussels sprouts 3g
- Carrots 2g
- Cauliflower 1g
- Collard greens 4g
- 1 cup raw baby spinach 1g
- Green beans 2g
- Mushrooms 2g

Heart-Healthy Fats

OILS

- Avocado oil
- Flaxseed oil (keep refrigerated and do not heat)
- Hemp oil (keep refrigerated and avoid high heat)
- Olive oil
- Sesame oil (keep refrigerated and avoid high heat)
- Walnut oil (keep refrigerated and avoid high heat)

OMEGA-3 FISH

- Atlantic mackerel (avoid king mackerel due to its mercury content)
- Rainbow trout
- Salmon
- Sardines

NUTS/NUT BUTTERS AND SEEDS

- Almonds and almond butter
- Brazil nuts
- Cashews
- Chia seeds
- Flaxseed
- Macadamia nuts
- Pecans
- Peanuts and peanut butter
- Pine nuts
- Pistachios
- Sunflower seeds
- Walnuts

MISCELLANEOUS

- Avocado
- Low-sodium olives

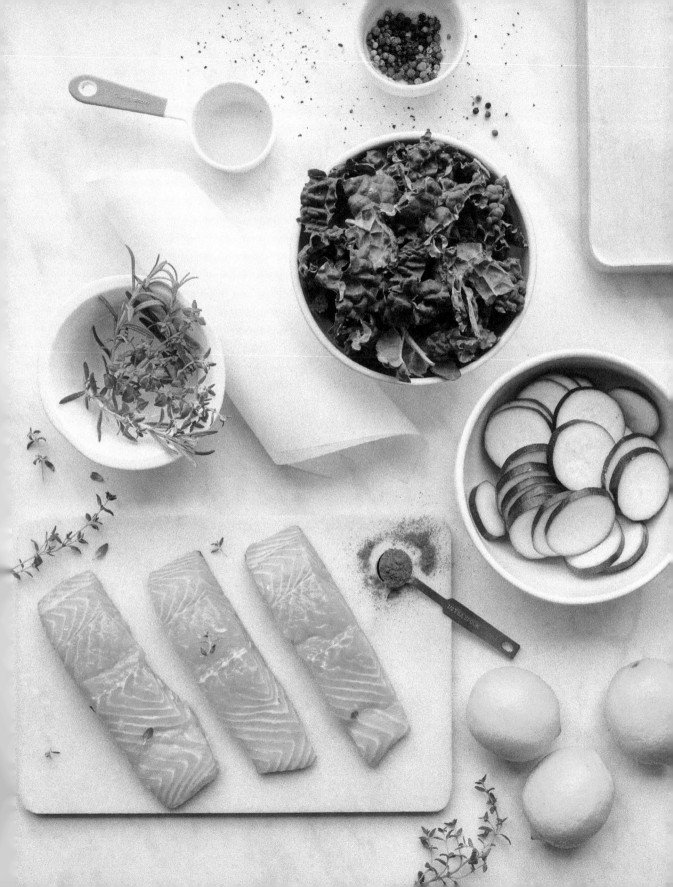

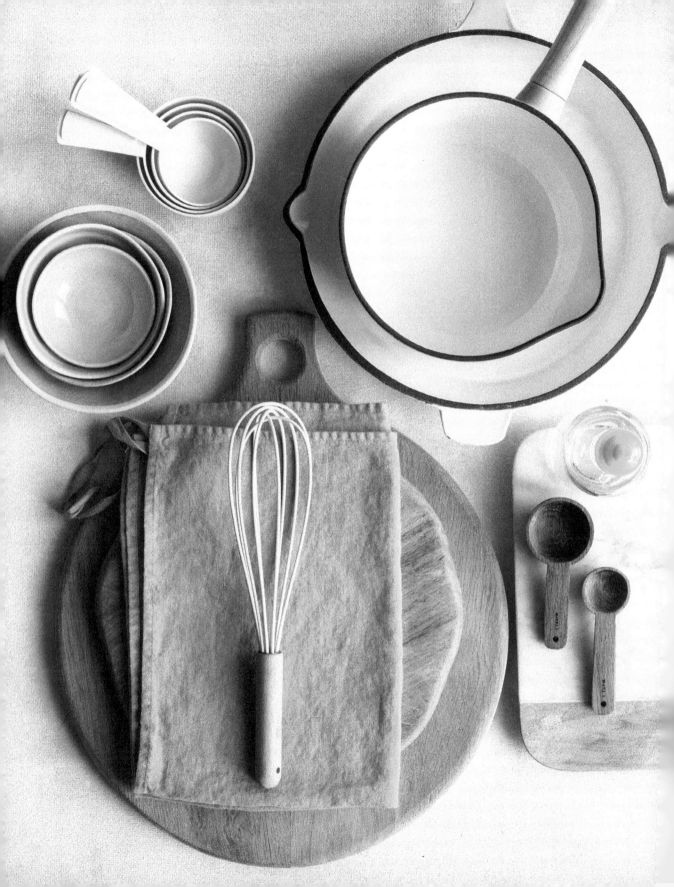

Measurement Conversions

	US STANDARD	US STANDARD (OUNCES)	METRIC (APPROXIMATE)
VOLUME EQUIVALENTS (LIQUID)	2 tablespoons	1 fl. oz.	30 mL
	¼ cup	2 fl. oz.	60 mL
	½ cup	4 fl. oz.	120 mL
	1 cup	8 fl. oz.	240 mL
	1½ cups	12 fl. oz.	355 mL
	2 cups or 1 pint	16 fl. oz.	475 mL
	4 cups or 1 quart	32 fl. oz.	1 L
	1 gallon	128 fl. oz.	4 L
VOLUME EQUIVALENTS (DRY)	⅛ teaspoon	——	0.5 mL
	¼ teaspoon	——	1 mL
	½ teaspoon	——	2 mL
	¾ teaspoon	——	4 mL
	1 teaspoon	——	5 mL
	1 tablespoon	——	15 mL
	¼ cup	——	59 mL
	⅓ cup	——	79 mL
	½ cup	——	118 mL
	⅔ cup	——	156 mL
	¾ cup	——	177 mL
	1 cup	——	235 mL
	2 cups or 1 pint	——	475 mL
	3 cups	——	700 mL
	4 cups or 1 quart	——	1 L
	½ gallon	——	2 L
	1 gallon	——	4 L
WEIGHT EQUIVALENTS	½ ounce	——	15 g
	1 ounce	——	30 g
	2 ounces	——	60 g
	4 ounces	——	115 g
	8 ounces	——	225 g
	12 ounces	——	340 g
	16 ounces or 1 pound	——	455 g

	FAHRENHEIT (F)	CELSIUS (C) (APPROXIMATE)
OVEN TEMPERATURES	250°F	120°F
	300°F	150°C
	325°F	180°C
	375°F	190°C
	400°F	200°C
	425°F	220°C
	450°F	230°C

Resources

American Kidney Fund's Advocacy Network (KidneyFund.org/advocacy)
Helps raise awareness and supports those living with kidney disease.

Cronometer (Cronometer.com)
A great website for tracking foods and analyzing recipes.

DaVita (DaVita.com)
Worldwide kidney healthcare company with patient resources, recipes, nutrient analyzer, and support networks.

Kidney Community Kitchen (KidneyCommunityKitchen.ca)
Information, resources, and recipes from the Kidney Foundation of Canada to help individuals manage their kidney disease and offer group support.

KidneyU (UKidney.com)
A leading resource for kidney disease information and resources.

Magic Kitchen (MagicKitchen.com)
Chef- and dietitian-created meals for a kidney-friendly diet.

Mom's Meals (MomsMeals.com)
Offers premade kidney-friendly meals with home delivery.

National Kidney Foundation (Kidney.org)
A leading health organization dedicated to fighting kidney disease and offering patient facts and resources on kidney disease in the United States.

References

National Institute of Diabetes and Digestive and Kidney Diseases. 2017. "What Is Chronic Kidney Disease?" www.niddk.nih.gov/health-information/kidney-disease /chronic-kidney-disease-ckd/what-is-chronic-kidney-disease.

National Kidney Foundation. 2021. "Kidney Disease: The Basics." www.kidney .org/news/newsroom/factsheets/KidneyDiseaseBasics.

US Centers for Disease Control and Prevention. 2021. "Chronic Kidney Disease in the United States." 2021. www.cdc.gov/kidneydisease/publications-resources /ckd-national-facts.html.

Index

Acknowledgments

Without the support and encouragement of my loved ones, publishing two cookbooks in a short time frame would not have been possible. Thank you for your stomachs while I tested recipes, but also for filling mine when I was working late.

About the Author

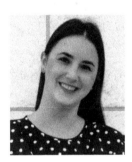

Emily Campbell, RD, CDE, MScFN, is a registered dietitian and certified diabetes educator with a master of science in food and nutrition. As the owner of Kidney Nutrition, she works with her clients in Canada to help those living with chronic kidney disease make nutrition and lifestyle changes to preserve kidney function. The author of *The Complete Renal Diet Cookbook*, Emily is passionate about making recommendations for foods that are both delicious and nutritious.

CPSIA information can be obtained
at www.ICGtesting.com
Printed in the USA
JSHW011908280122
22324JS00002B/2